CONQUERING
INSOMNIA

An Illustrated Guide to Understanding Sleep and
a Manual for Overcoming Sleep Disruption

Colin M. Shapiro, Ph.D., M.B., F.R.C.P. (C)

James G. MacFarlane, Ph.D., A.C.P.

Mohamed R.G. Hussain, M.D., C.C.F.P.

1994
Empowering Press
Hamilton, Canada

Printed in Canada
by Remarque Communications

ISBN 0-9695171-3-0

To Joy, Kathy, and Shehnaz who have tolerated, usually with good humor, the sleep-disruptive effects of having husbands who, in the course of their medical training and sleep research, have not always kept the most sociable of hours; and in tribute to the late John Cleghorn, one of the early Canadian sleep researchers.

Contents

PART III: HOW TO DEAL WITH INSOMNIA

APPENDIX   118

GLOSSARY   119

PREFACE

Insomnia is a very common symptom which in most cases is transitory. If it recurs or becomes chronic it can be a most troublesome and disruptive problem. It is no exaggeration to say that some of the most distressed patients we have treated are patients suffering with insomnia. Far too often it is treated trivially.

If insomnia is dealt with sensibly, problematic insomnia and its chronic aspects can often be avoided. Requisites for preventing acute insomnia from becoming chronic insomnia are tackling the problem thoughtfully and fully when it first appears. It is not usually simply a matter of taking medication but also involves a change in behavior. For many individuals this change is not made easily — witness the difficulties people have losing weight or stopping smoking.

The purposes of this book are to give information about sleep and to provide a manual of things to do and ways in which to change one's behavior to achieve a more normal sleep pattern.

The objective of improving the sleep of patients with insomnia is three-fold: immediate relief from the sense of tiredness that may be associated with insomnia, a decrease in the risk of a variety of medical illnesses associated with insomnia, and insurance in terms of better sleep later in life.

Behavior cannot be changed simply by reading a set of instructions and then applying them. If this were possible, you could simply read a book about how to play golf and directly anticipate becoming a pro. This clearly does not occur. Changing behavior requires practice of the new behavior. This is best done by carefully adapting current behavior to a more desirable pattern and shifting the routine of behaviors that may be disrupting sleep.

We believe that for more than 90 percent of people with insomnia the specific cause and solution will be dealt with in these pages.

Professor Colin M. Shapiro
J.G. MacFarlane
Dr. M.R.G. Hussain

ACKNOWLEDGMENTS

We are most grateful for the assistance of Marjorie Fleming, Honorie Pasika, and Stephanie Neprily in preparing the text. We thank Alison Harkin, Claudette Messier, and Elizabeth Stacey for figures. We thank Sari O'Sullivan for producing many of the original illustrations, and Ann Newton for her meticulous editing. To our publishers, who had reservations about our proposed deadlines, we give thanks for their skepticism and productivity. Finally, we thank Deena Sherman for providing some of the original photographs.

Grateful acknowledgment is made for permission to reprint previously published material: excerpts from *Oxford Dictionary of Quotations,* 3rd ed., Oxford University Press, 1979. Reprinted by permission of Oxford University Press.

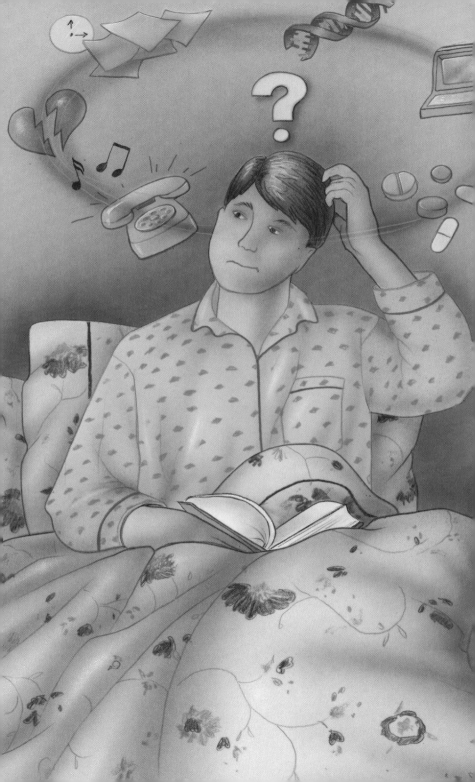

CHAPTER ONE

What is Insomnia?

What is insomnia? Is it a difficulty in falling asleep? Is it interrupted sleep or an inability to maintain sleep once you have fallen asleep? Or is it sleep that's just not long enough or good enough to refresh or rejuvenate you in preparation for the next day?

Any of the above conditions may be true of insomniacs. Your life may become complicated by the frustrations of sleeplessness. Fatigue, irritability, drowsiness, and sleepiness occur during the day with deteriorating capacity to function. Your personal relationships may suffer. It is quite possible to experience both sleep onset and sleep maintenance insomnia. Whatever the complaint, people with chronically disturbed sleep become vulnerable to addiction to drugs which promote sleep, or to alcohol. Both may aggravate their sleep problem and diminish their general well-being. Often, because of their personalities and temperament, these people are more concerned with problems in their daily lives, perceive more responsibilities, carry a greater sense of guilt, and are overly occupied with their ambitions.

We all complain about sleeplessness at some time in our lives. Usually we realize this is transient, brought on by an incident, illness, or stress which we often keep to ourselves. With adequate rest, a healthy diet, and healthy state of mind we recover when the event which caused it passes. The recovery may take days or weeks. When it goes beyond this period, we may become trapped in a downward spiral where the fear of not sleeping becomes the source of anxiety which causes the insomnia.

It is important to recognize that there is a considerable degree of normal variation in sleep duration and that many factors, e.g., age and sex (chapter 4) influence sleep. Normal variation in sleep length should not be confused with insomnia.

At 40 years of age, 7 percent of the population experience insomnia. At age 70 about 35 percent suffer with insomnia. Females are more affected at this age and about 40 percent of them regularly take some sleep-inducing prescription medication.

Adults generally sleep six to ten hours a night. Some people have a normal, uninterrupted sleep of from three to six hours a night. They are alert in the morning and function normally in their daily tasks. They are considered "short sleepers" and have no underlying disorder.

"Long sleepers" may require ten to 12 hours of sleep to wake up alert and function well the next day. "Long sleepers" may be unhappy with less sleep. Daytime alertness (i.e., a lack of drowsiness) is a good indicator of adequate sleep. Test yourself. If you can lie down at any time during the day and fall asleep in less than five minutes, you probably did not have enough sleep the preceding night.

Another variant which may be confused with insomnia is a shift in the biological clock to an earlier or later time (chapter 4). This shift of the clock forces some to sleep earlier in the evening while others cannot fall asleep until the early hours of the morning. The former may be considered early birds or "larks" and the latter night persons or "owls". A popular misconception about insomnia is that if you go through a period where your sleep has been poor, even for one night, you may think you have to "make up" the lost sleep. That is, you will require more sleep the following night. This is simply not true. In fact, a teenager named Randy Gardener still holds a world record achieved by remaining awake for almost 11 consecutive days without sleep. When he finally did go to sleep, he slept for 17 hours and awakened feeling fully refreshed. Clearly he did not even begin to make up the hours of sleep he had lost. However, in this catch-up sleep, the sleep depth and quality may be greater so that the restorative effect of this sleep is more than simply a reflection of its duration.

Insomnia is common in many medical (including psychiatric) conditions. This will be discussed in later chapters. (Figure 1-2)

IS INSOMNIA A MODERN EPIDEMIC?

A recent American study showed that approximately one-third of those surveyed reported some type of sleep disturbance. Here are some highlights from the most recent community-based survey data on insomnia including those from a recent Gallup poll:

Epidemiology
- 36% of the population occasionally suffer from some sort of sleep disturbance.
- 10 to 15% of the population describe the problem as serious.
- Less than 20% of patients with insomnia ever discuss it with their doctors.
- 80% of visits to a family doctor for insomnia are related to an emotional crisis.

- Daytime naps become more frequent and longer with increasing age.
- All insomnia-related symptoms are more common in females.

Sleeping Pills
- 60% of insomniac patients who see their doctor are currently taking sleeping pills.
- 45% of these patients are chronic users of sleeping pills.
- A recent large study has shown that some sleeping pills are more likely to be associated with longer use. At the top of the list were Oxazepam (Serax) and Triazolam (Halcion).
- Sleeping medications are the most commonly prescribed class of prescription medication.
- An independent research group calculated that the average Halcion user in 1989 took that drug for periods of 148 to 296 days (five to ten months).

Figure 1-2

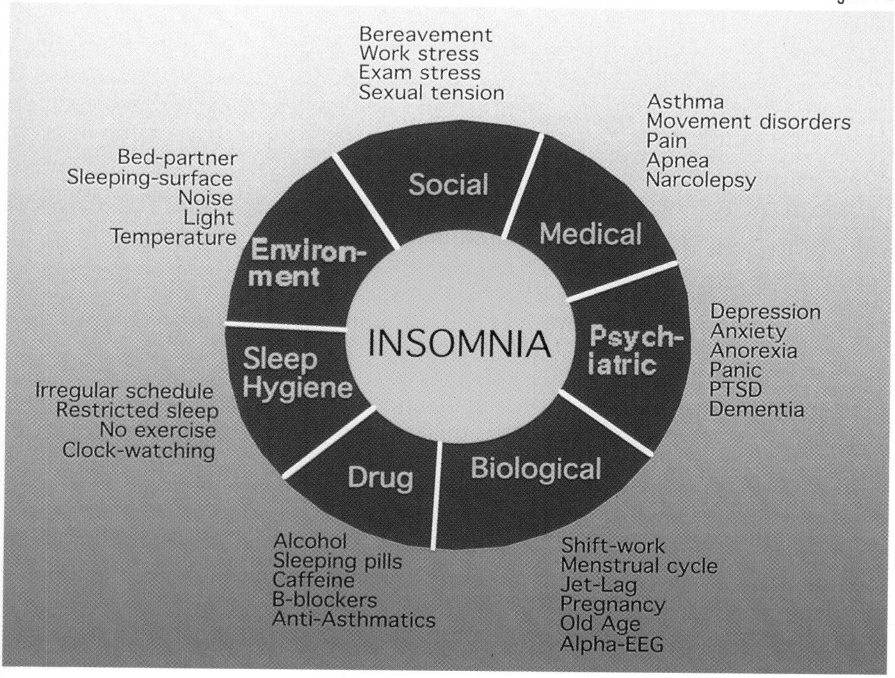

Type of Sleep Problem
- 56% of insomniacs have difficulty initiating sleep.
- 67% wake up in the middle of the night.
- 57% have problems getting back to sleep after waking up.
- 72% report waking up in the morning feeling drowsy or tired.
  (Some people with insomnia have more than one problem.)

Dangers
- In the United States, two hundred thousand auto accidents per year are caused by drowsiness.
- Insomniacs are more than twice as likely to report vehicle accidents in which fatigue was a factor.

These facts alone show that insomnia should not be treated trivially.

Social Problems
- There is a significant deterioration in the quality of life for the insomniac including impaired concentration, memory, ability to accomplish daily tasks, and enjoyment of interpersonal relationships.
- The ability to cope with minor irritations is significantly impaired in people with chronic insomnia.
- 10% of insomniacs report falling asleep while visiting friends.

Other Issues
- 40% of insomniacs self-medicate with over-the-counter medications or alcohol.
- 66% of insomniacs report that they do not have an understanding of available treatments.
- The tendency to seek medical advice increases with age.

These are but a sampling of the statistics on the impact of disturbed sleep on individuals and society.

Is insomnia a modern epidemic? The answer appears to be unequivocally - YES. The so-called "Toronto syndrome" of long working days with long commuting times leading to a restriction of sleep time (getting up early to miss the traffic) is clearly a 1980s and 1990s phenomenon leading to daytime fatigue and increased use of stimulants such as coffee. Symptoms of insomnia diminish the quality of life by reducing participation in, and enjoyment of, many everyday activities that non-insomniacs take for granted. The symptoms of insomnia, including increased daytime sleepiness and fatigue, increase the risk of accidental physical injury. The long-term effects on general health and life expectancy show a clear increase in both disease and early death in short sleepers.

What is Sleep?

Blessings on him who invented sleep, the mantle that covers all human thoughts, the food that satisfies hunger, the drink that slakes thirst, the fire that warms cold, the cold that moderates heat, and, lastly, the common currency that buys all things, the balance and weight that equalizes the shepherd and the king, the simpleton and the sage."

(Miguel de Cervantes, 1547-1616, Don Quixote)

Sleep is one of the most fascinating activities that seems to be common to all living organisms. It is a state of consciousness that is distinct. Dreaming is part of sleep but very distinct from deep restorative sleep and, almost certainly, it has a different function.

Are we in control of our actions and responsible for our behavior when we sleep or dream? Do we know if animals dream? Why do dolphins sleep with one half of their brain at a time? Why do king penguins sleep in large groups standing up? Why do survivors of major traumatic experiences adapt better to it over their life-times if they suppress their dreams? These questions and many others intrigue scientists and add to the rich web of information we have about sleep. Many aspects of this daily process remain a mystery.

When a person cannot sleep, certain questions arise: What is sleep? What is the function of sleep? What happens if I don't sleep? These are the questions addressed in the first section of this manual.

"I slept like a log" is probably the most popular metaphor used to describe sleep of "exceptional quality". The log, supposedly like the well-rested sleeper, remains horizontal, motionless, and lifeless throughout the night. However, this is an inadequate description of sleep. You can sleep sitting up. Movement during sleep is normal and perhaps essential, and some brain and body functions reach their highest level of activity during sleep. To explore and understand sleep, you must appreciate its counterpart, wakefulness. Certain brain centers are responsible for actively maintaining wakefulness. Figure 2-1 shows a cross-section of the brain. Think of it as a cauliflower.

The green stalk and stems of the cauliflower are below and within each "head". These green portions are similar to the brainstem. The white flower is folded and elaborated upon the end of each stem so that most of the green portion is hidden from view. These white portions are similar to the cortex of the brain.

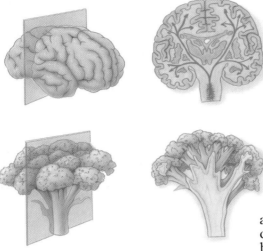

The cortex is the "thinking" part of the brain, which allows us to remember, decide, plan, express, create, as well as calculate and initiate body movements. So, what else do you need? It would seem as if the cortex does it all. But without the brainstem, the cortex is virtually stranded. The brainstem connects the cortex to the body while regulating, molding, and perfecting incoming and outgoing messages. It receives direct signals from the body, interprets them, and then sends modified signals to the cortex. The brainstem is also able to tell the cortex when it is time to search for food and water, when it is time to fight, when it is time to have sex, and when it is time to lie down and sleep.

Figure 2-1
The brain and the cauliflower

The brainstem also plays a vital role in keeping the cortex "awake" or vigilant. A series of centers within the brainstem and a network of nerve fibers projecting to the cortex act collectively to stimulate cortical activity. Thus, we are able to remain awake as long as there is adequate stimulation of the cortex by the brainstem.

What is it to be "awake"? What are you experiencing? In a global sense, the answer is quite straightforward. You are awake as long as you maintain sufficient cortical activity to keep you in direct contact with your external environment. You are attentive to certain cues such as sight, smell, and sound, each of which elicits a set of responses. During wakefulness you know what is going on around you and can react accordingly (shown by the arrows in Figure 2-1).

However, the longer you remain awake, the greater the pressure or need to sleep. A group of researchers at Harvard and the University of Tennessee have shown that if you keep a goat awake and then collect the cerebrospinal (brain) fluid of the sleeping goat and inject it into an awake rabbit, the rabbit will quickly go into a deep sleep. In addition to the involvement of the nervous system in sleep, there is a chemical/hormonal/sleep substance which perhaps builds up during wakefulness, promotes sleep, and then is dissipated by sleep.

The transition from wakefulness to sleep is heralded by physical and mental signs of sleepiness and fatigue. These include

Figure 2-2
A person being prepared for a sleep recording

decreased vigilance, reaction time, and problem-solving ability, and increased emotional reactivity (i.e., irritability). These are vital considerations for the sleepy driver. Sleep is actually an active process and the brainstem is once again the driving force.

Other specific areas of the brainstem become increasingly active at the end of a period of wakefulness. Nerve fibers from sleep generating centers terminate at the wakefulness centers and inhibit them. These sleep centers actually inhibit the activity of the wakefulness centers such that as the sleep centers become more active, the wakefulness centers become less active. The overall effect is a reduction and termination of the "wakefulness drive" to the cortex. At some point in this process sleep ensues.

Sleep can be conceived of as an altered or different state of consciousness. It is not a state of *un*consciousness. During sleep we do not attend fully to our external environment, yet some very interesting internal events are unique to sleep.

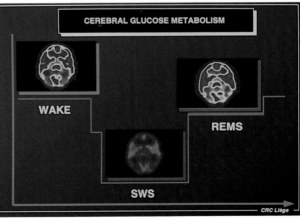

Figure 2-3
Brain metabolism differs in different sleep stages

If someone is hooked up to a physiologic recorder (a polysomnograph) to document events which occur during sleep (Figure 2-2) it becomes evident that sleep is divided into particular stages. The two main divisions are deep (restorative sleep) and rapid eye movement sleep (REM or dream sleep) (Figure 2-6).

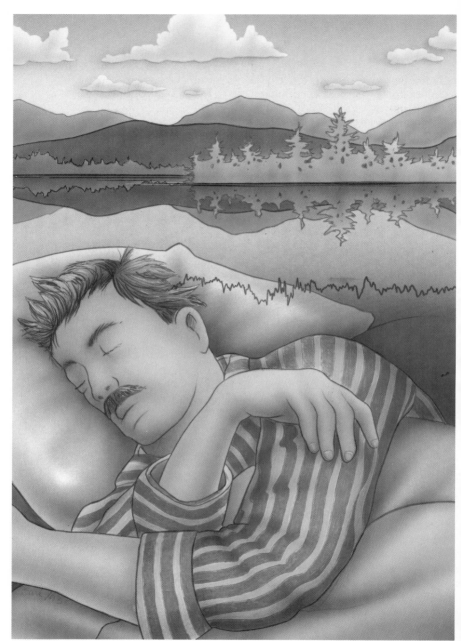

Figure 2-4
Different brainwave
patterns reveal
the type of sleep
a person is having

8

REM Sleep

    Fantastic events occur during REM sleep. Brain metabolism is increased (sometimes exceeding that when awake) (Figure 2-3), and muscle tone is decreased so much that if you go to sleep in a chair, you will fall out of the chair after entering REM, unless you awaken to catch yourself! A small group of cells in the brain inhibit motor activity during dream sleep. These cells are found in the locus coeruleus. In 1965, a French sleep researcher was able to show that destroying these few cells in cats would lead to their "acting out their dreams", for example, licking a plate of milk that was not there. It is because of the activity of these cells that we do not act out our dreams. Other features of dream sleep include rapid eye movements (REM) and body twitches. The next time someone comments that your cat or dog appears to be chasing a rabbit in his sleep, you can tell them that your pet is in REM sleep.

Another curious factor of REM sleep is penile erections in the male. If a man is awakened from REM sleep he will invariably have an erection. There is no evidence that these erections are related to sexual excitement or dream content. Doctors sometimes use this feature of sleep to differentiate between impotence of psychological or physiological origin. If the problem is physiologic there will be no nocturnal REM-related erections.

Dreams

By far the most exciting aspects of REM sleep are the wild, funny, disjointed, surreal, scary, and vivid dramas which play in our heads most often during REM. A day-dream is merely a thought or memory. Hearing and/or seeing things that are not really there during wakefulness is considered a hallucination. Seeing and/or hearing things during sleep is a dream. The content of dreams alters in response to aging, conflict, sexual identity, stress, and psychopathology. Dreams are in color, occur in real time, and become longer and more frequent in the second half of the sleep episode (Figure 2-5). When dreams become disturbing they are known as nightmares and can interfere with sleep.

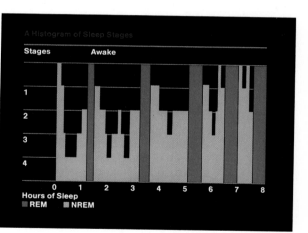

Figure 2-5
The alternating stages of sleep follow a pattern through the night

"Thoughts, words, and deeds, the Statute blames with reason; But surely Dreams were ne'er indicted Treason."

(*Intro. to Robert Burns's,* "A Dream")

Sleep Stages

NonREM sleep can be divided into four separate stages based almost exclusively on brainwave patterns. Stage I is considered the transition between wakefulness and sleep. The transition through Stage I into Stage II constitutes a successful passage into sleep. Approximately 50 percent of the nocturnal sleep is spent in Stage II sleep. Stage III and IV are generally lumped together as slow wave sleep or deep sleep. The brainwaves during these stages are much slower (lower frequency) and larger (higher voltage) than any other sleep stage (Figure 2-6). More effort is required to awaken a person from slow wave sleep than any other stage, thus the term "deep sleep".

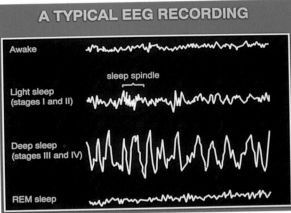

Figure 2-6
Different brain wave patterns in different sleep stages

Sleep is a relatively orderly process. Sleep architecture refers to the relative duration of each sleep stage and the timing of its occurrence during the sleep period. Generally we start off in Stage I sleep, and progress through stages II, III, and IV over a ninety-minute period before entering REM sleep. At the end of the REM episode another ninety-minute cycle begins. A restful sleep depends as much on appropriate sleep architecture (including sleep continuity) as it does on the actual total amount of sleep obtained. Nine hours of sleep which is fragmented and disturbed will not be as restorative as seven hours of solid sleep. As the brain detects that an adequate sleep has been attained, the activity of the sleep generating centers begins to wane thereby allowing increased activity of the wakefulness centers, and normal waking function is restored.

What is the Function of Sleep?

ost people have some idea of the functions of the heart and lungs and other bodily systems. However, even most physicians could not give a clear and coherent explanation of the function of sleep. If they were to say that it is simply to "give some rest", they would not be able to back it up in any specific way.

There have been many theories regarding the function of sleep. These include the idea that sleep is a time when daytime problems are sorted out, or memories are sifted or consolidated. Other theories have suggested that sleep plays a protective role by removing an organism from an unsafe environment to which it is not properly adapted. Alternately, it may play a more passive role by providing a time when the body is not active and one is simply absolved from consuming food and storing energy because one is expending less energy.

There is, however, one theory where a large jigsaw of evidence can be put together to make a clear case which explains sleep function. This is the *restorative theory of sleep*. Many would say that their grandmother knew that sleep was a restorative time, but in the scientific and medical community this was not widely accepted until very recently.

If you want to understand problems associated with insomnia, it is imperative to understand the function of sleep; only then will you fully appreciate the benefits of correcting your insomnia and the importance of a normal sleep pattern. In thinking of insomnia, one needs to consider that sleep has both a quantitative (i.e., how much sleep we have) and a qualitative component (i.e., how good is the sleep that we have). We have already remarked on the different types of sleep. The restorative theory suggests deep sleep (slow wave sleep) possesses the most restorative properties.

The following sections describe the "pieces of the jigsaw" that have helped us put together the puzzle of sleep function. Sleep serves a restorative purpose and therefore a great deal of emphasis should be placed on having normal sleep, both in terms of *amount* of sleep and *quality* of sleep.

11

Growth

"Jock, when ye hae naething else to do, ye may be ay sticking in a tree; it will be growing, Jock, when ye're sleeping."

(Sir Walter Scott, 1771-1832, The Heart of Midlothian)

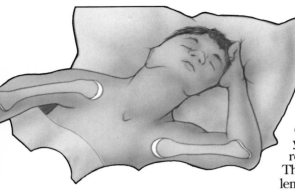

If sleep is restorative, then one would presume that sleep is a time when growth occurs. A variety of research studies suggest this is the case.

The first and most obvious experiment would measure growth during the day and during the night. Some years ago, a group of Dutch researchers did exactly that. They accurately measured bone length, both in the morning and at

Figure 3-1
Bones lengthen at night

night, in a group of adolescent subjects (Figure 3-1). They found that each night the adolescent would grow a little and each day there would be a slight shrinkage of bone length with net growth overall.

Another aspect of growth is the release of a growth hormone. For many years it had been known that there were a variety of triggers that would promote growth hormone release. These included exercise and a protein meal. A team of Japanese researchers established that growth hormone rises dramatically in the blood stream shortly after sleep onset (Figure 3-2).

Figure 3-2
The brain releases growth hormone during sleep

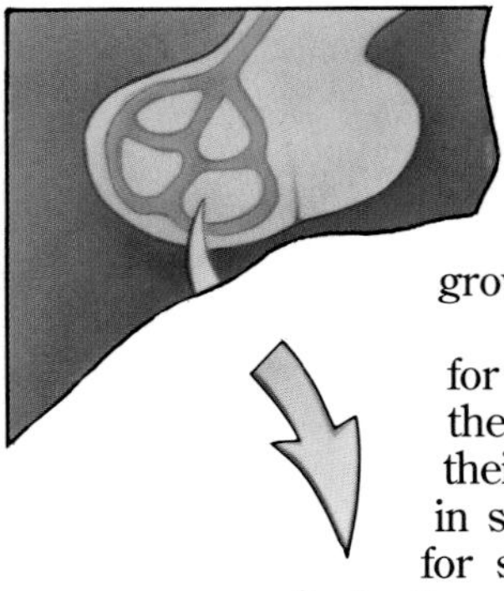

Subsequent research has shown that this growth hormone release occurs particularly in association with the first episode of slow wave sleep and that there is a second peak, often in association with the second slow wave sleep episode, during the night. The obvious implication is that there is a linkage between the periods of slow wave sleep and growth hormone release and, thereby, with growth.

We have shown that when people are extra tired, for example, after being deprived of sleep for one night, they have increased growth hormone release during their catch-up or recovery sleep (Figure 3-3). Conversely, in some situations, those experiencing sleep disruption for some specific reasons, may exhibit an absence or diminution of growth hormone release. People who are excessively dependent on alcohol are one example. They may have normal amounts of slow wave sleep, but there is no associated growth hormone release. This indicates a qualitative

12

problem in their sleep, even if the quantitative components are present. Children who have been severely abused occasionally exhibit "psychosocial dwarfism": they have stunted growth as a result of sub-normal nocturnal growth hormone release. It has been shown that cells divide most rapidly during sleep irrespective of the time of day that a particular animal sleeps (Figure 3-4).

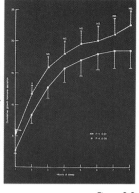

Figure 3-3
Young, healthy men release growth hormone early in the night and more so after sleep deprivation

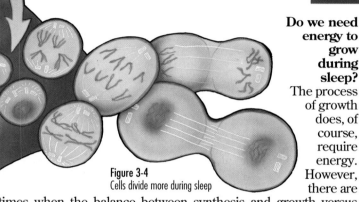

Figure 3-4
Cells divide more during sleep

Do we need energy to grow during sleep?
The process of growth does, of course, require energy. However, there are times when the balance between synthesis and growth versus breakdown and activity are tipped in favor of breakdown. One example is the sprinter running a 100 meter dash. The runner would be taking in a great deal of oxygen and breathing heavily (oxygen providing part of the energy that the body uses). During the following night he would experience a drop in energy utilization. This can be established by direct measurement (calorimetry) or by measuring how much oxygen is used at any given time. Oxygen consumption decreases during the night in part because people are keeping still, lying down, and not eating food, exercising or doing other things requiring energy. Oxygen consumption is even lower if a person is asleep while lying down during the night, and is lowest during deep sleep (Figure 3-5). Although this may seem a paradox, it is with the drop in oxygen utilization that maximal growth and restoration occurs.

Figure 3-5
Lower energy and oxygen use during sleep tilt the balance in favor of restoration

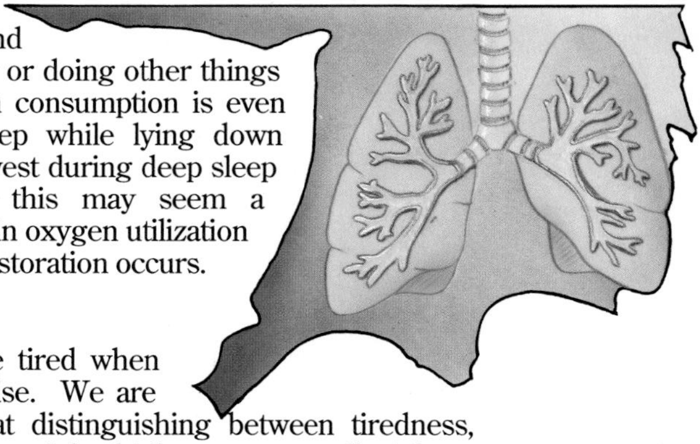

Exercise and Sleep

Many of us feel more tired when we have done some exercise. We are generally not very good at distinguishing between tiredness, sleepiness, and fatigue. We might think any one or all of these

13

Figure 3-6
Energy expenditure by day leads to more restorative sleep

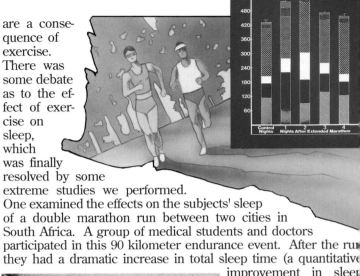

are a consequence of exercise. There was some debate as to the effect of exercise on sleep, which was finally resolved by some extreme studies we performed. One examined the effects on the subjects' sleep of a double marathon run between two cities in South Africa. A group of medical students and doctors participated in this 90 kilometer endurance event. After the run they had a dramatic increase in total sleep time (a quantitative improvement in sleep amount). They also had a doubling of the amount of deep or slow wave sleep (an increase in the qualitative aspect of their sleep) (Figure 3-6). This dramatic increase in deep sleep tapered off over three to four days.

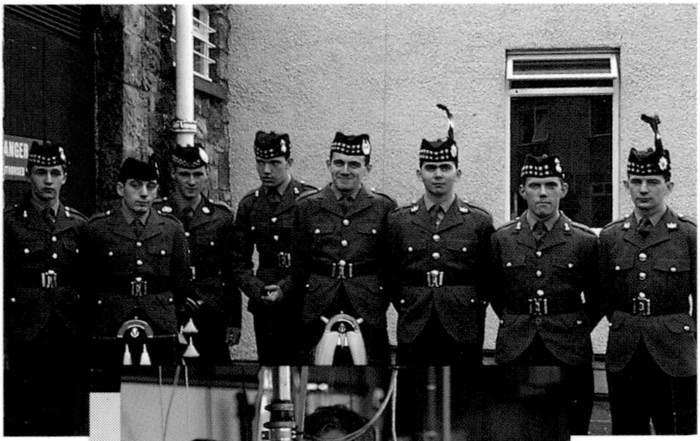

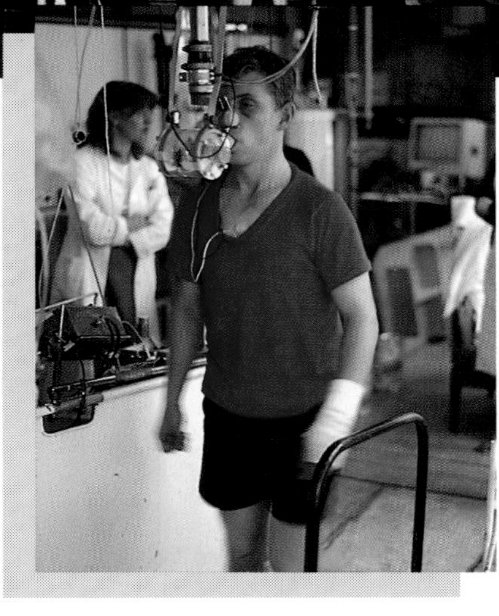

Figure 3-7
Fitness facilitates sleep

A man who tried to break the world walking marathon record stayed awake for seven days and six nights, and was on his feet for more than 98 percent of that time. He walked 334 miles and his name was entered in the *Guinness Book of Records*. When his sleep was studied for three days after this exploit, his slow wave sleep was extensive and there was also a very large amount of growth hormone release.

There is an orchestration of sleep effects which occur after exercising. The more extreme the exercise, the greater the degree of

14

sleep changes. However, there comes a point when the strenuousness of the exercise is so extreme that pain and disruption of sleep begin to occur. Too much exercise for a given level of fitness may disrupt sleep.

Scottish army recruits who had both their fitness level and their sleep measured at three points in their basic training showed that as they got fitter the quality of their sleep improved (Figure 3-7).

Weight Gain and Sleep

Anorexia nervosa is a condition, most commonly found in young women, where there has been the intentional loss of weight to below normal levels. When these people are refed there is an increase in deep sleep associated with the rapid body growth that occurs during this time (Figure 3-8).

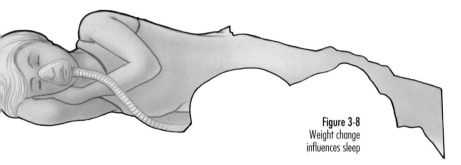

Figure 3-8
Weight change
influences sleep

Clinical Sleep Studies

People who are less active (e.g., patients who are blind, or suffer from some form of paralysis) have less deep sleep than normal. Less activity during the day means less need for deep restorative sleep at night.

People with increased thyroid activity (Figure 3-9), resulting in a faster body metabolism, have an increased amount of deep sleep, whereas patients with low levels of thyroid hormone who often are perceived to be slow, sluggish, and sensitive to the cold, have lower levels of deep sleep.

A number of drugs alter the composition of sleep. For example, a drug used as an appetite suppressant (fenfluramine) increases body metabolism and also increases deep sleep (Figure 3-10).

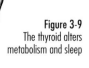

Figure 3-9
The thyroid alters
metabolism and sleep

These clinical studies support the notion that sleep is linked to metabolism and is restorative.

15

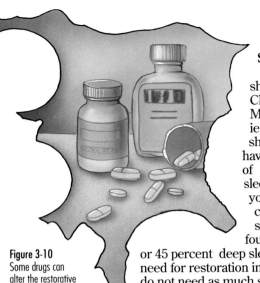

Figure 3-10
Some drugs can alter the restorative aspects of sleep by altering metabolism

Sleep Disruption

There are a number of famous short sleepers including Winston Churchill, John F. Kennedy, and Margaret Thatcher. Research studies on people who have sleep of short duration have shown that they have a disproportionately large amount of deep sleep. In most people sleeping seven or eight hours as a young adult, there will be a sleep component of 20 percent deep sleep; but those who sleep three or four hours will often record up to 40 or 45 percent deep sleep. They are likely satisfying their need for restoration in a more efficient way and therefore do not need as much sleep (Figure 3-11).

Deprived of sleep on a single night, you will likely have increased deep sleep the subsequent night. This indicates that a "need" or "debt" for deep sleep has built up over the preceding 36 hours of wakefulness.

Figure 3-11
A short sleep episode contains a greater proportion of restorative sleep than a long sleep episode

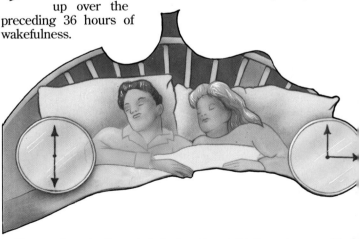

If your sleep is disrupted during the night there is more likely to be a deep sleep episode in the latter part of the night after the sleep disruption. Also the size of the large slow waves in this deep sleep grows. This again indicates qualitative as well as quantitative aspects of sleep. This deep sleep episode is also more likely to be associated with another growth hormone peak.

Most deep sleep occurs early in the night. This is a further indication that deep sleep is essential. As sleep progresses lighter sleep is more plentiful and, toward the end of the night dreaming sleep tends to predominate (Figure 2-5).

Developmental Studies (Figure 3-12)

Sleep is not always the same at different stages of life (chapter 4). As one progresses through life, the amount of deep sleep gradually diminishes.

During adolescence there are a number of hormonal changes which lead to growth and the acquisition of secondary sexual characteristics. Often adolescents are berated because they stay in bed all day and "sleep too much". However, their bodies are simply responding to the need for growth by increasing the amount of sleep.

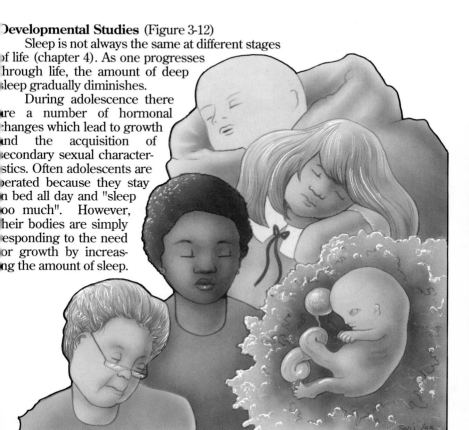

Figure 3-12
A greater proportion of restorative sleep occurs during the growing phase of life

Animal Studies

Sleep studies on animals have shown a relationship between metabolic rate and sleep. (Figure 3-13).

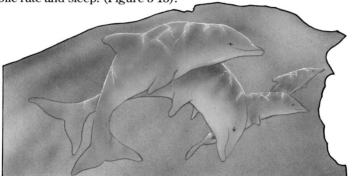

Figure 3-13

If sleep is restorative, then having the right amount and the right type of sleep are important in overcoming any sleep difficulties. Many sleep clinics and laboratories offer detailed measurement of sleep quantity but there are very few situations in which the quality of sleep is assessed adequately.

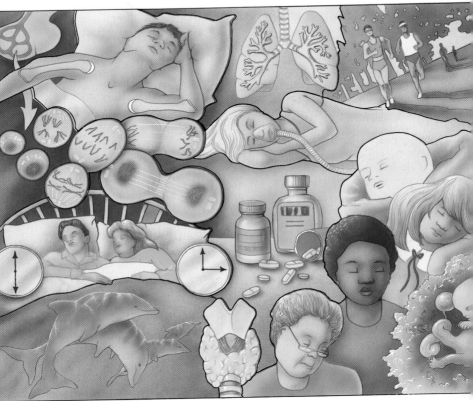

Figure 3-14
All of the different pieces in the complex jigsaw puzzle, individually shown in this chapter, come together to support the theory that sleep serves a restorative function

Influences on Sleep

Age and Sleep
As one gets older sleep patterns change. A newborn infant sleeps on average 16 hours a day; a person in his 20s might sleep eight hours a day; someone in her 40s seven hours a day; and someone in his 70s may sleep only six hours daily. Not only does the total amount of sleep change, but the composition of sleep changes dramatically (Figure 4-1). A newborn spends half the sleep time in dreaming sleep, whereas by adulthood this is down to one-fifth or one-quarter of sleep time.

Figure 4-1

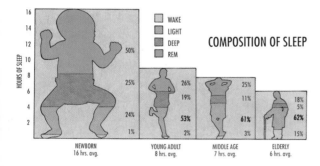

COMPOSITION OF SLEEP

The other striking change in sleep that occurs as one moves from young adulthood to old age is the dramatic decrease in deep sleep. We consider this the most restorative component of sleep and it is probable that this decline in deep sleep leads to complaints of feeling unrefreshed and unrestored. For example, in a young adult approximately 20 percent of her sleep time is deep sleep. Between the ages of 20 and the mid-forties deep sleep declines to approximately 10 percent of sleep time. By age 70 only 5 percent of sleep time is deep sleep. We think this may be linked to the development of memory loss and dementia in the elderly. This decline is also one possible reason for the increased demand for sleeping pills by the middle-aged and elderly. It follows that medications that suppress deep sleep (most benzodiazepines and other older sleeping pills) may have harmful effects, whereas hypnotics which increase deep sleep may be of specific benefit.

Aspects of deep sleep decline in the elderly. For example there is less growth hormone release and the large slow wave which are characteristic of deep sleep become smaller.

Another difference occurring with age is that the elderly spend more time in bed. This in itself may cause disruption of sleep — it is as if the body is thinking that it has more time to have its sleep and, therefore, does not consolidate sleep. The net effect may be sleep interrupted by frequent awakenings. These awakenings cause a sensation of fatigue the next day, possibly leading to daytime napping and a consequent decrease in sleep drive the following night.

Dreaming sleep remains relatively constant throughout adulthood. Its decline is often a prelude to intellectual deterioration.

Numerous other changes occur with age. Snoring becomes more common. Approximately 60 percent of men and 45 percent of women in their 60s snore. In the elderly it becomes fairly common to have occasional apneas during sleep (chapter 16) whereas in individuals under the age of 60, one rarely finds more than five respiratory disturbances per hour of sleep. In the elderly almost half may have a significant number of apneas each night. Approximately 30 percent of individuals over the age of 6 have periodic limb movements during sleep.

There may be changes in circadian (± 24 hour) rhythms. In dementia, for example, there may be a total breakdown of circadian rhythms with the elderly being active during the night and sleeping during the day, causing considerable family disruption. Occasionally, a relief admission to hospital with more brightly lit environment and more social interaction may help resynchronize their circadian rhythms.

Having the right perception of what kind of sleep is reasonable and normal as we age goes a long way to ease our concerns about sleep patterns.

Diet and Sleep

As children we are told to eat the proper foods, that certain things are good for us, and to drink our milk before we go to bed. These articles of traditional wisdom are often ignored. Like adequate sleep, proper eating habits are essential for good health. Certain foods may even influence our sleep.

Lack of food leads to metabolic changes which may make us restless in our sleep, and may lead to awakening. Extreme starvation can depress the central nervous system into hypoglycemic coma.

Eating a meal rich in carbohydrates can promote sleep. This may occur through release in the digestive tract of such hormones as cholecystokinin which induce sleep.

Going to bed hungry is not a good habit, nor is having the evening meal at different times. This upsets our biological rhythm which may contribute to insomnia. Avoid going to bed immediately after a heavy meal. Your digestive mechanisms are very active then and indigestion could disrupt your sleep.

It is claimed that obese people appear happier and sleep better; thinner people are often characterized as being anxious and sleeping less; but the relationship between weight and sleep is complex and has not been sufficiently studied.

Tryptophan, an amino acid abundant in dairy products, eggs, meat and nuts, has been shown to induce sleep.

Calcium deficiency causes muscle irritability and cramps. Young children, pregnant women, and the elderly often require more calcium to relieve cramping which occurs especially at night. Warm milk which offers plenty of calcium and tryptophan promotes a better night's sleep especially when taken regularly.

Numerous commercially available products claim to promote a better night's sleep. Most of these (e.g., Ovaltine, Horlicks) contain cereal and milk products. They contain some of the important ingredients mentioned earlier. They are also high in calories.

For improved sleep many advocate drinking camomile tea in the evening. The Chinese take ginseng and orange juice mixed with honey, the Pueblo Indians eat mushrooms, the Burmese eat pollen cake, and the English claim an apple chewed slowly before bedtime helps sleep.

Do not make a habit of eating after awakening during the night. You may inadvertently train your body to awaken you from sleep anticipating food.

Gender Effects on Sleep

Normal sleep patterns differ slightly in men and women and these differences depend, in part, on age. The decline in deep sleep related to age occurs ten years earlier in men. Females in their 30s find that they take a long time to go to sleep, but have a longer sleep time.

There are many sleep disorders which vary in relation to gender. Women more commonly experience hypnotic dependent sleep disorder, adjustment sleep disorder, nocturnal leg cramps, restless legs syndrome, and psychophysiological insomnia. Sleep disorders more frequently observed in men include: obstructive sleep apnea, central sleep apnea (this equalizes after menopause), rhythmic movement disorder, sleep terrors, and enuresis. Sleep paralysis is one of a number of conditions which have no sex differentiation.

A number of theories have been put forward to explain why women may have more insomnia including the possibility that women have more disrupted sleep associated with child rearing and, therefore, have worse sleep in later life. This is contradicted somewhat in laboratory studies in which women have slightly better sleep quality in middle age. Twice as many women as men take sleeping medications. It may be that male physicians choose to deal with female complaints of sleep disruption this way. An alternative explanation is that women have more psychiatric illness which may lead to more insomnia and more prescriptions for sleeping pills. Finally, it may be that sleep disruption in older women is partly a consequence of menopause and a perceived change in the subjective quality of sleep that comes on abruptly. It may be that symptoms of menopause, such as hot flashes and other factors, disrupt sleep in middle-aged women and lead to increased use of hypnotics.

Sleep in Pregnancy

Many factors influence sleep in pregnancy. It is a period of clear growth in terms of the fetus and placenta. There is also an increase in the vascular load on the body causing increased bladder filling at night, particularly in the last trimester. The need to urinate clearly disrupts sleep. The large abdominal mass and associated discomfort may also lead to a disturbance of normal sleep. Sequential recordings of the sleep patterns of pregnant women show a progressive rise in the amount of deep sleep (Figure 4-2). This deep sleep is related to increased energy costs.

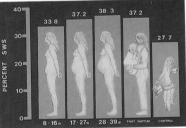

Figure 4-2

There are marked endocrine changes during pregnancy. There are rises in estrogen, progesterone, prolactin, and cortisol. All of these hormones have slightly different effects on sleep.

The timing of childbirth has a considerable impact on subsequent development of the "blues". A recent study was carried out showed that women who had their labors and gave birth during the day were far less likely to develop the blues than women who had a major sleep disruption by having labor or childbirth at night (Figure 4-3). These observations again emphasize the importance of normal sleep patterns and the potential hazards of disrupted sleep. The increase in fatigue that many women describe in the first and third trimesters may be somewhat different. The former may be more related to growth whereas the latter may be more related to dragging a heavy load around all day.

Effects of the Menstrual Cycle on Sleep

At menopause a woman's sleep quality deteriorates. Studies

show that replacement estrogen decreases the amount of wakefulness that occurs during sleep, but there are no consistent findings as to how the menstrual cycle alters sleep.

In the mid-1960s, one researcher found an increase in dreaming sleep in the premenstrual period. However, the subjects were taking a variety of medications which possibly invalidates the research. In the early 1970s, a study of only three women suggested that there is an increase in deep sleep in the premenstrual period. In 1980, another study found that there is a decrease in deep sleep during the menses. A recent study group of eight women showed an increase in Stage III sleep near ovulation and most wakefulness in the premenstrual phase of the cycle.

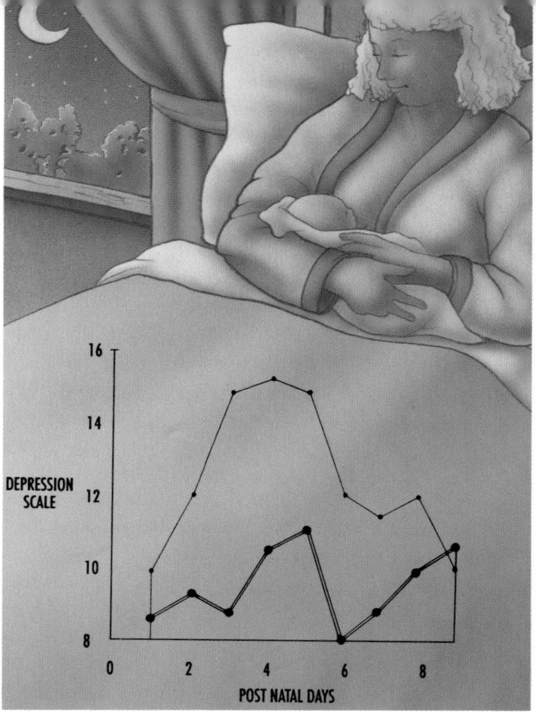

This study also compared sleep in women with premenstrual depression to those with no symptoms. The depressed women had more light sleep and less dreaming sleep and their temperatures dropped early in the night.

Figure 4-3
The thin line charts post natal "blues" in women who had babies at night, while the double line shows women giving birth by day

Biological Rhythms/Shift Work

Two modern-day inventions have made the most notable differences in the way humans spend their waking time — electric light and television. Artificial light allows you to carry on into the night as if it were daytime; television provides the excitement and stimulation that promotes the postponement of other activities including sleep. Most North Americans turn on their lights and televisions with the onset of darkness, and turn them off only when they are compelled to go to bed.

Animals that are awake during the day and asleep at night are referred to as diurnal. Those that sleep by day and have their waking period during the night are nocturnal. For diurnal animals living in their natural habitat, the onset of darkness is their biological cue that it is time to lie down and sleep. Intuitively, it seems unlikely that an animal so perfectly in sync with its environment would have problems with insomnia or excessive daytime sleepiness.

Humans are constantly adjusting their biologic rhythms to suit their needs. The biological rhythm affecting sleep is called

23

the circadian rhythm. Partying all night, extended work hours, shift work, and air travel across several time zones all disturb significantly the normal relationship between the biologic clock and the natural environment. The disruption of this clock may lead to insomnia.

Your own biologic clock resides in the brain approximately two inches behind your eyes. This bit of brain tissue, about the size of a pea, is the Suprachiasmatic Nucleus (SCN). It detects incoming light information from the retina and transforms it into biologic time signals which are sent to all parts of the body. This brain clock is able to keep the body and mind apprised of the time, day, month, and the time of year. This helps the body to schedule sleep and wakefulness, the menstrual cycle and, in lower animals, the seasonal cycles of reproduction and hibernation.

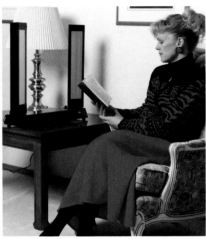

The most powerful time cue for human biologic rhythms appears to be the twenty-four-hour light/dark cycle. While the absence or presence of light can be converted into biological signals, more subtle cues, such as light intensity and absolute duration, can provide seasonal information. This is the basis for bright light phototherapy (Figure 4-4), for seasonal mood disorders (seasonal affective disorders - SAD), and for sleep onset insomnia.

We have shown in humans that it is possible to induce sleep and resynchronize circadian rhythm using the natural hormone melatonin. This hormone, which is released from the pineal gland, is the biological mediator of light/dark information which lets the whole body know the time of day.

Figure 4-4

Other signals to the clock are the timing of food intake (mealtimes) and social cues. Regular eating habits can assist internal time-keeping and even arriving for work every morning can be an important synchronizer.

If a human or lower animal is placed in an environment free of external time cues where information regarding the time and day or night is obscured (clocks and watches removed, access to television and radio denied) the SCN clock keeps on "ticking". It continues to provide time information for conscious activities — a time to wake up, a time to go to bed, and a time to eat. As well, it coordinates the timing of other cycles that cannot be appreciated consciously such as rhythms of hormone secretion and nerve cell regeneration. If a person is kept in a time-free environment for ong enough, the biological clock eventually begins to drift out of phase. When he is brought back into his natural environment, his biological rhythms and the environmental rhythms will be out of sync. This may well give rise to initial symptoms of insomnia and excessive daytime sleepiness.

People placed in underground caves where they received no cues as to time (light, clocks, mealtimes) and were simply left to "free run" lived in cycles from a twenty-five-hour day up to a fifty-hour day.

What stops us from following our natural rhythm? The answer is Zeitgeibers. Zeitgeibers are the external factors which reset our rhythms to twenty-four hours. These may be social activity, work schedules, alarm clocks, mealtimes, and light and dark changes. Humans exhibit a great variation in their reactions to different Zeitgeibers. There are thus wide differences between individuals in their abilities to fall asleep, wake up, and function alertly during the day.

As a general rule, the more you react *consistently* to Zeitgeibers, sticking firmly to regular hours, the easier it becomes for your inner clock to follow suit.

One common problem resulting from a lack of routine is the difficulty you may have getting up for work or school on Monday morning. With the freedom that you feel on weekends in the absence of time constraints typical of a normal work week, the temptation is to disregard normal cues for bedtime and wake-up time. By the time Monday comes around, your biological clock is still delivering messages to your brain and body that there is time to sleep when the alarm goes off at 7:00 a.m. Furthermore, when you try to get into bed on Monday night at normal weekday hours, your brain may still perceive that it has several hours of waking left before bedtime. At this point, you are in a state of phase delay. All biological rhythms have shifted to a later time with respect to your external environment. For some, complete recovery from this phase delay pattern will not come until midweek. This implies that normal timekeeping occurs only on Thursday and Friday, after which the pattern of phase delay begins again.

Sometimes you have no choice in the selection of a perfect schedule to meet the needs of your natural biological rhythms. When you step off a jet traveling east or west, you can expect that your mind, body, and wrist watch are still indicating the time it is back home, which will be several hours out of sync with the social and environmental time of your destination. Thus, mealtimes, sleep times and wake up times are completely disrupted. If one is traveling to deliver a vital presentation at a business meeting or to partake in Olympic competition, this desynchrony is of great concern. The traveler may find his mind alert, his reaction time quick, his decision-making acute, and his physical energy at its highest point, just at the time when all those around him are preparing to retire for the night. At that important meeting at 11:00 a.m. the following morning, although the people around him have the highest expectations of his performance, his biological clock is still delivering messages to his brain and body that it is time to lie down and sleep (Figure 4-5).

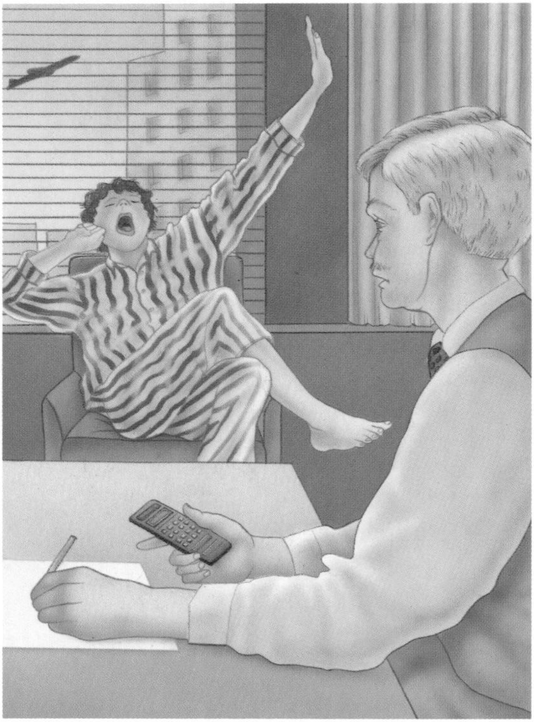

Figure 4-5

Disruption of the clock can be somewhat more insidious. In the non-stop, twenty-four-hour urban environment, people at work and people at leisure can easily ignore messages from their biologic clocks as well as those from their natural environment. Students stay up and study for exams, workers extend their working days, and others get caught up in the excitement of the constant stream of entertainment coming from their television sets until late in the evening. There is a potential to become "jet lagged" within your own bedroom. A vicious cycle may ensue. People extend their day into the late evening or early morning hours, attempt to awaken in order to get to work on time the following day, and arrive at work in a state of mild sleep deprivation. Feelings of fatigue and sleepiness may build up to the point that daytime naps are required even while at work. Studies have shown that 15 percent of workers nap sometime during the day while at work. Napping during the day may, to some extent, compensate for the sleep debt, allowing the person to once again extend his waking hours. When he attempts to break this pattern either on expert advice or upon the realization that his restricted sleep is having a negative effect on his daytime performance, he may find that when he gets in bed at a normal time, he is unable to sleep. This completes the vicious cycle. The choice of a late bedtime has now become the rule rather than the exception. Breaking the cycle may be an ordeal taking several nights of tossing and turning.

What Happens if You Do Not Sleep Normally?

his chapter concentrates on the nature of insomnia and addresses the question, "Does it really matter?"

There are many definitions of insomnia. The word comes from the Latin *somnus* meaning sleep. We provided and prefer the definition in the *Cambridge Encyclopedia*: "unsatisfactory sleep, whether in quantity or in quality. It may be a component of a variety of physical or mental disorders. There may be difficulty in either initiating or maintaining sleep, a preoccupation about sleep, and interference with social and occupational functioning as a result of sleep disruption".

You can see that there are many different dimensions to insomnia. There are issues of quality and quantity of sleep and of degree and frequency of sleep disruption. There is also the issue of the effects of this disruption on daytime functioning. Finally, two individuals may sleep for the same length of time, but their depths of sleep may differ dramatically. In an extreme example, one individual might have no sleep every Saturday night and complain bitterly of this occasional insomnia; whereas, another person might have a change in sleep duration from seven hours of sleep each night to five hours, every night of the week. The complaints of these two individuals might differ widely as well as the effects on their overall performances. The former may have a particularly bad Sunday because of fatigue, but be able to work reasonably well during the week. Whereas, the latter may have chronic performance difficulties and irritability throughout the week and weekend. The impact of all of these different aspects of insomnia will be touched on in this chapter.

It is important to make an estimation of the severity of your insomnia as treatments for varying degrees of insomnia differ. For a person who has relatively mild or very occasional insomnia a treatment strategy which emphasizes behavioral techniques will usually be sufficient. For someone with very severe insomnia it is usually necessary to control the insomnia initially with medication. While this artificial control is obtained, the individual should be working on behavioral techniques so that when the catalyst of the hypnotic medication is removed, the quality of sleep continues to be as good as, or nearly as good as, when he was taking medication. In some circumstances the behavioral techniques are better learned without taking medication.

Mild insomnia occurs on an almost nightly basis. The individual receives an insufficient amount of sleep or does not feel rested after the usual sleep period. There is usually little or no damaging impact on social or occupational functioning. There may be irritability, some daytime anxiety or fatigue, tiredness and perhaps a feeling of general restlessness intended in part to combat the feeling of sleepiness.

Moderate insomnia occurs every night. The individual does not have a sufficient amount of sleep or does not feel well rested after the usual amount of sleep. This may be the result of poor sleep quality. There is some degree of impairment of social and/or occupational function. There are always sensations of restlessness, mild anxiety, tiredness, and daytime fatigue, and invariably some degree of irritability.

Severe insomnia also occurs nightly. There is a marked impairment of occupational and social functioning. There is always a sense of not being fully alert, some daytime fatigue and tiredness. Irritability is invariably present, as well as a degree of anxiety.

You can see that these categorizations are on a continuum. It is not possible to say that a certain level of sleep disruption produces specific consequences. Many people will describe a couple of bad nights of sleep after which their bodies feel achy and painful. Some people who have chronically poor sleep complain of marked muscular pain and a sensation of physical weakness. Some of these individuals would be described as suffering from fibrositis or chronic fatigue syndrome. It may be that at a certain level of sleep disruption the impact on the immune system is such that they are more susceptible to infection and more likely to develop chronic pain disorders.

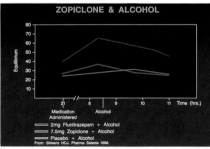

Conversely, an individual who has some reason for daytime fatigue whether it is insomnia or the consumption of alcohol, may have a dramatic worsening in his daytime functioning with the addition of a second factor to increase his fatigue level. For example, some sleeping medications (but not others), when added to alcohol, have a cumulative effect on daytime sleepiness (Figure 5-1). This is a multiplicative effect. This example indicates that the impact of sleep disruption depends on factors other than simply the effect of sleep alone.

Also, certain drugs cause daytime sedation. The impact of these sleeping medications differs in people of different ages. The

Figure 5-1
Avoid alcohol when taking medication

older the individual, the greater the daytime effects of using sleeping pills. Paradoxically, a larger proportion of old people take sleeping pills.

Quantity of Sleep

There is a normal amount of sleep that an individual has at any particular point in his life cycle.

A typical sleep recording generates a paper record approximately half a kilometre long. It must be analyzed, in 20-second segments, for the whole of the night (Figure 5-2). As a consequence the number of individuals studied to establish these norms is relatively small. It is possible to learn what the normal amount of sleep is for any one individual. In addition, we have also discovered the normal range of dreaming and non-dreaming sleep at any particular age, the average time taken to fall asleep, and numerous other features of sleep architecture typical for a person of a particular sex, at a particular age.

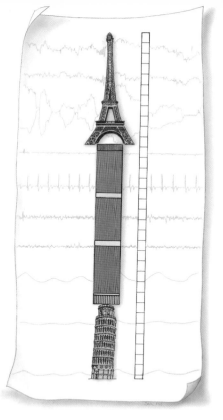

If a person who normally sleeps for six hours sleeps for only three it is easy to see that she is suffering from insomnia. However, if a person who normally sleeps for nine hours sleeps for only six she may have just as many problems in terms of daytime function as the former. Absolute duration of sleep is not the only factor determining the impact of insomnia.

Figure 5-2
A one-night sleep record is as long as the Eiffel Tower, World Trade Center, and Leaning Tower of Pisa stacked one on top of the other

For many insomniacs studied in the sleep laboratory there is a subjective under-reporting of the duration of sleep compared to laboratory findings. Many physicians are aware of this and will treat patients with insomnia as either neurotics or complainers. It is our view that many such individuals are indicating that they have poor *quality* of sleep. Clinical experience tells us that if we rephrase the issue for the insomniac and say, "Does it feel as if you have only five hours of sleep?" (when the objective measures indicate seven hours of sleep duration), the insomniac will often say, "Yes, that's how it feels". It is the *subjective* perception of sleep disruption that is most important. This discrepancy in many cases relates to a poor quality of sleep for which physicians and sleep researchers have little in the way of measures and understanding. Occasionally, a person will be adamant that they do, in fact, sleep very little or not at all. This is a specific problem which will be discussed later.

29

Nonrestorative Sleep

There are many different reasons why sleep may be nonrestorative (Figure 5-4). We describe subsequently conditions in which a person has either repeated leg movements or apneas during the night which cause a disruption of his sleep, although not awakening him fully. Such individuals often complain of daytime fatigue and sleepiness. This can be easily understood. Most people who have this problem are subjectively unaware of their sleep disruption.

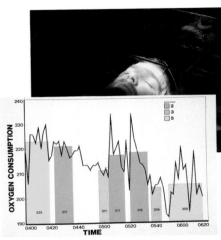

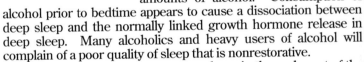

It is well established that people who are depressed or have insomnia have a higher level of oxygen consumption during the night than normal. This raised level of oxygen consumption may be an indicator of nonrestorative sleep (Figure 5-3).

Recall that during sleep there is a dramatic release of growth hormone early in the night. Notable exceptions are patients who consume excessive amounts of alcohol. Consumption of alcohol prior to bedtime appears to cause a dissociation between deep sleep and the normally linked growth hormone release in deep sleep. Many alcoholics and heavy users of alcohol will complain of a poor quality of sleep that is nonrestorative.

Figure 5-3

During sleep body temperature drops in the early part of the night. There is considerable debate as to whether sleep causes or facilitates this decline or whether the change in temperature facilitates the onset of sleep. Either way, in situations where a temperature decline does not occur, individuals will often complain of a nonrestorative sleep. People who have traveled from Canada to Japan have a temperature rhythm which is 12 hours out of sync with their customary day and night sleep rhythm. Rather than being on a falling part of the curve when one would be inclined to go to bed, say at midnight, their temperature is rising. Often sleep during this time of high temperature will be described as poor and nonrestorative.

In our sleep clinic we have seen people with chronic fatigue referred for assessment of their sleep or patients with various aches and pains referred often to rheumatologists with a diagnosis of fibrositis. In such patients with pain, it is common to see a specific alteration in sleep pattern. In normal individuals, before going off to sleep and when their eyes are closed, there is a characteristic alpha brain wave pattern. Usually, as the person drifts off to sleep, this alpha pattern disappears until they awaken. However, in patients with fibrositis particularly, it is common to see brief bursts or long stretches of this alpha pattern occurring within the sleep period. At present, we know of no good biological reason for this. The doctor may say, "It is as if you are partially awake when you are asleep". Clearly this is a contradiction in terms. Many patients will spontaneously respond, saying that this is exactly how they feel, and will then elaborate by saying something like, "It is as if I am just skimming below the surface of sleep", or "I feel my sleep disruption causes me the pains that I suffer". There is clearly an acknowledgment of the interaction between their sleep and their body pain. In such individuals, nonrestorative aspects of their sleep may be contributing to their medical condition. It is impossible at present to tell whether or not it is the pain causing the sleep disruption, or vice versa. Experiments have shown that if one takes a group of normal individuals and subjects them to disrupted sleep they are more likely to develop a variety of aches and pains.

The preceding examples indicate some factors that may lead to a poor quality of sleep and to non-restorative sleep. An individual with some of these disorders will show no abnormality on a standard sleep laboratory recording. One of the challenges of the next few decades in sleep research is to devise ways of measuring sleep quality, as well as sleep amount. A further challenge is separating out problems of fatigue, tiredness, and sleepiness which may be partly dependent on amount of sleep, as well as quality of sleep.

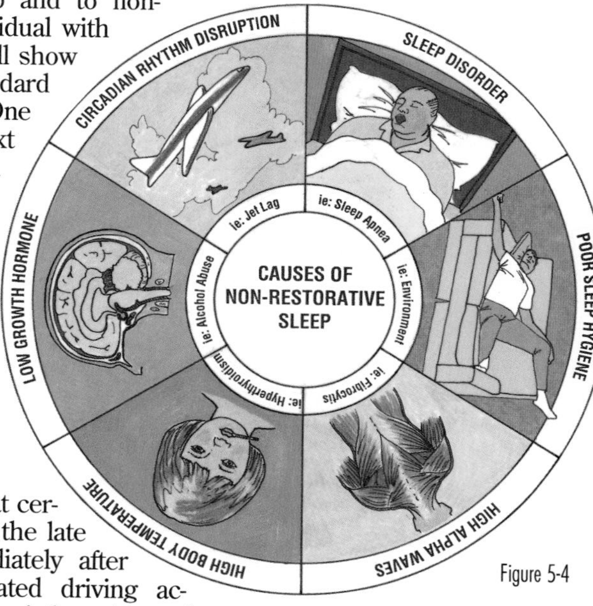

Figure 5-4

"Dangers of Sleep"

People die most often at certain times — either toward the late sleeping periods or immediately after awakening. In fatigue-related driving accidents, there is a circadian variation with peaks at approximately 3:00 a.m. and 3:00 p.m. (Figure 5-5). Sleep may be a dangerous time. Lack of sleep may have important consequences.

A number of large studies have shown that individuals who have unusually short sleep are more likely to die at an earlier age. Yet, obviously, disease may be killing the person, as well as caus-

31

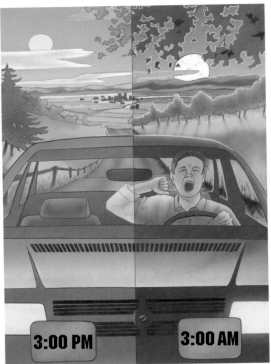

3:00 PM　　**3:00 AM**

Figure 5-5
The headlights
highlight the
times of
maximum fatigue

ing his sleep disruption. However, even taking into account statistical risks for heart disease, strokes, diabetes, high blood pressure, exercise, smoking, physical health, alcoholism, and weight, the effect of short sleep on mortality still stands. Even among the elderly, in whom sleep duration is usually shorter, those who sleep exceptionally short amounts are more likely to die earlier. There is also evidence that people who have short sleep are more likely to have heart attacks.

A large study in Finland demonstrated a clear association between poor sleep and poor subjective health. Restless sleep occurs in patients with a variety of medical disorders including rheumatoid arthritis and chronic kidney disease. Persons with multiple sclerosis do not complain of restless sleep more than the average patient of a family practitioner, but they will often complain of pronounced fatigue.

The number of accidents and major disasters that occur as the result of sleep deprivation highlights the danger of insomnia. There has been considerable debate about the problems of the sleep-deprived junior hospital doctor who may make mistakes in treatment. There is also concern about the possible effects of sleep disruption and excessive fatigue on pilots brought on either by jet lag or long working hours. The consequences of sleep disruption are obvious.

A young mother with small children has repeated sleep disruption, whether she is breast feeding or simply answering the nighttime needs of restless children. The effects, in terms of damaging long-term sleep patterns and short-term irritability, have had little study. It is possible that long periods of poor sleep during one part of your life may have consequences many years later. Shift workers who have switched to straight days have been shown ten years later to still have more disrupted sleep than people who never worked shifts. The implication may be that when you are young you might appear to tolerate sleep disruption from a variety of causes, but as you age and your sleep system is less robust, the consequences of those earlier indiscretions may come back to haunt you.

C H A P T E R   S I X

A Sleep Diary to Help You Assess and Rate your Sleep

We are now ready to help you to discover *your* usual sleep pattern and to evaluate your daytime behavior as it may affect your sleep. You will document your level of fatigue and tiredness before going to sleep and your level of alertness and sense of refreshment on waking. At the end of this exercise you will be able to look at the possible interrelationship between your sleep pattern, your daytime activities, and your subjective feelings about being refreshed.

Each of two people get four hours sleep. One may be in bed for five hours, getting into bed, switching off the light within a few minutes, taking 20 minutes to fall asleep, remaining solidly asleep for four hours and then lying awake in bed for perhaps half an hour on awakening in the morning (Figure 6-1).

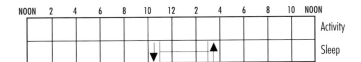

Figure 6-1

The other may get into bed at 10:00 p.m., take two hours to fall asleep, then sleep in half-hour bursts with half-hour wakeful periods between sleep episodes for the next five hours, and have a last hour of solid sleep waking to an alarm clock set for 6:00 a.m. (Figure 6-2).

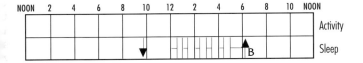

Figure 6-2

The sense of alertness and also of frustration that these two people have might be very different, yet both have had four hours of sleep. The first person may simply be a regular short sleeper or be restricting his sleep. A short sleeper would feel alert after four hours of sleep, but someone who is restricting his sleep is likely to have daytime fatigue. The second person may have consumed a large amount of alcohol or caffeine which may have contributed to his disrupted sleep; whereas, he normally might sleep six or seven of the eight hours he is in bed.

We would like you to record your sleep over a one week period. It is *important* that you cover a *full* week.

The diary on pages 36 and 37 asks you to record: the day; the date; if you took a pill; the time you got into bed; the time it took you to fall asleep (please do not watch the clock to establish how much time it takes); the number of times you woke up during the night; the time you finally woke up at in the morning; and if you used an alarm. Both you and an observer looking at your chart will be able to establish the continuity of your sleep, how difficult it is for you to fall asleep, whether you are, perhaps, spending too much time in bed, and a number of other important factors relating to insomnia. Fill out this chart each morning and evening.

You are required to record daily activities. For example, if you have two drinks of alcohol at 7:00 p.m. with dinner, you would record the information as follows (Figure 6-3).

Figure 6-3

NOON	2	4	6	8	10	12	2	4	6	8	10	NOON	
			AA										Activity
													Sleep

If at the middle of the day you had an hour of exercise and then had a light snack you would record the information as follows (Figure 6-4).

Figure 6-4

NOON	2	4	6	8	10	12	2	4	6	8	10	NOON	
X S													Activity
													Sleep

34

If you got into bed at 1:00 a.m., fell asleep at 2:30 a.m., got up to use the bathroom at 5:00 a.m., got back into bed and slept until your wake-up alarm at 7:00 a.m., you would record the information as follows (Figure 6-5).

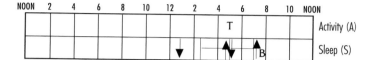

Activity (A)

Sleep (S)

Figure 6-5

In the diary on the following two pages, the right hand page records activities from the day after the night described on the left.

The chart on the left hand page provides a twenty-four-hour time frame.

Please complete these charts as you read the book.

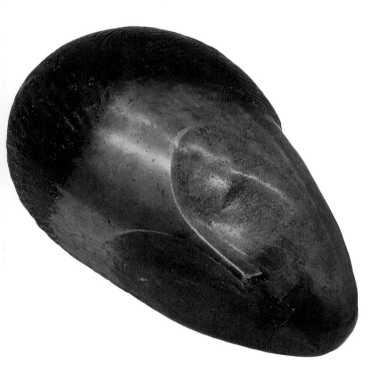

Figure 6-6
Carving of a
sleeping head

SLEEP AND ACTIVITIES RECORD

Instructions: It is important that you fill out this chart each evening
Mark your diary in the following way

ACTIVITIES
A - each alcoholic drink
C - each caffeinated drink: includes coffee, tea, chocolate, cola
I - interaction of calmness. This may be an exciting movie on TV, sexual
    intercourse before sleeping, a noise during sleep, or anxious thoughts
P - every time you take a sleeping pill or tranquilizer
P2 - every time you take any other pill
M - meals
S - snacks
X - exercise
T - use of toilet during sleep time

SLEEP TIME (including naps)
D - lights out/dark   Note each entry to bed with ↓
I - lights on/illumination   Note each exit from bed with ↑
B - alarm clock wakening   Note time asleep with ├────┤

| NOON | 2 | 4 | 6 | 8 | 10 | MIDNIGHT | 2 | 4 | 6 | 8 | 10 | NOON |

In the assessment of performance we would like you to use the scale from 0 to 10. For example, you might record a 1 or 2 if you are very sleepy, but if very refreshed, you would record an 8 or 9. This page is divided into two parts, those features that should be recorded 15 to 20 minutes after "arising" (A, B, C, D, E) and those items to be recorded before bedtime (1, 2, 3).

AWAKE - ZZZ CHART

Remember to complete A-E approximately 15 -20 minutes after awakening.
Complete 1-3 prior to switching off your light at night.

	Very Sleepy 0 1 2 3 4 5 6 7 8 9 10 Fully refreshed							
	Morning				**Evening**			
Fill in date under day	A	B	C	D	E	1	2	3
	Hours of sleep last night	I awoke very sleepy = 0; very refresh-ed = 10	I feel fuzzy headed = 0; alert = 10	My sleep was restless = 0; tranquil = 10	My sleep was better than usual = 0; as usual = 5; very dis-rupted = 10	I feel very tired = 0; wide awake = 10	I feel phys-ically worn out = 0; re-laxed = 10	I feel tense = 0; calm = 10
Monday								
Tuesday								
Wednesday								
Thursday								
Friday								
Saturday								
Sunday								

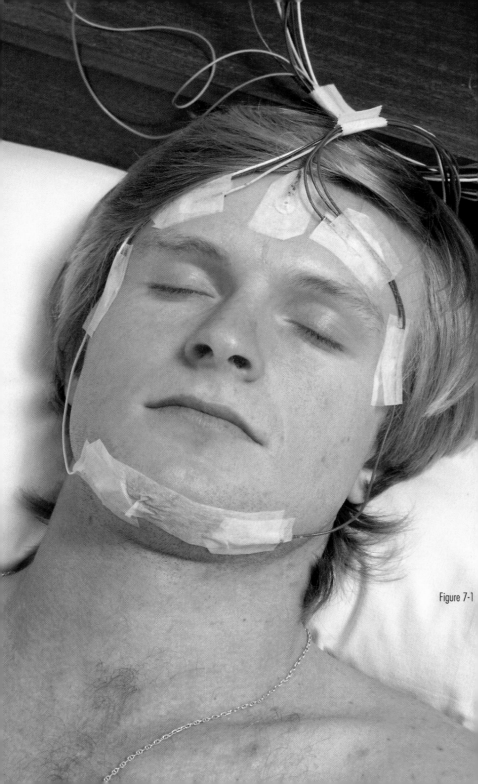

Figure 7-1

Sleep Laboratory Measures of Sleep

P eople who complain of chronic sleep disruption are often referred to specialized clinics offering expertise in sleep and sleep disorders medicine and facilities for overnight sleep studies and tests of daytime sleepiness.

About half of the people referred to a sleep disorders clinic require overnight study in a sleep laboratory. The "clinic" is the entire operation including physicians from a variety of clinical specialties and allied health professionals — psychologists, occupational therapists, and EEG technologists.

Sleep studies employ specialized equipment to monitor a variety of biological functions. Referral to the clinic is usually through your family doctor. Your first visit to the clinic will include a thorough medical consultation of approximately 30 to 60 minutes, completion of sleep and mood questionnaires, and possibly a physical examination. Information gathered in this visit will help determine whether an overnight study is needed. Often, behaviorial modification may be suggested to improve your symptoms. Medical factors contributing to your sleep problem may be discovered. A follow-up appointment will be made to assess the success of the behavioral, medical, or psychiatric intervention prescribed.

If there is no improvement at this point, or if a primary sleep disorder is suspected, an overnight sleep study will be scheduled, usually for one or two nights. If significant daytime sleepiness is also a problem, additional daytime testing may be required. Here are some of the most commonly asked questions about the sleep laboratory and their answers.

When Will I Stay in the Sleep Lab?

Most sleep studies take place during your normal sleep time. People on permanent night-shifts may be scheduled during the day. Most people report to the lab at 8:00 p.m., are "hooked-up" (Figure 7-1) between 9:00 and 10:00 p.m., and retire around 11:00 p.m. Sleep studies are terminated between 6:00 and 8:00 a.m. unless daytime testing is required. Each person sleeps in a single room as shown in Figure 7-3.

What Will Be Measured?

This will depend on the specific problem. A full-scale sleep study will measure: brain wave activity (electroencephalograph or EEG) from two electrodes or leads on the scalp; eye movements (electro-oculograph or EOG) from two leads placed at the outer corner of each eye; muscle tone (electromyograph or EMG) from two leads placed on the chin; leg movements (leg-EMG) from leads placed on the lower legs; heart rate (electrocardiograph or ECG) from two leads on the chest; breathing (respiratory effort) from elasticized belts, around the chest and abdomen; and oxygen concentration in the blood measured painlessly by a light sensor worn over the finger tip. Other measures for specialized problems include video recordings (for sleep walking) or measures of penile erections, with a device placed around the penis, for impotence investigations.

What Will This Show?

These recordings will generate a half-kilometer of tracings. Interpreting such a huge amount of data is no small task. Your record will be scored by a technician or sleep specialist for the following information: how long you slept; how well you slept; amount of deep sleep; amount of dream sleep; movements during sleep; sleeping positions; breathing during sleep; heart rhythms; snoring; apneas (pauses in breathing); leg movements; brain wave activity (e.g., alpha rating). These data, along with your medical history, allow the specialist to determine whether you have one of 88 specific sleep disorders.

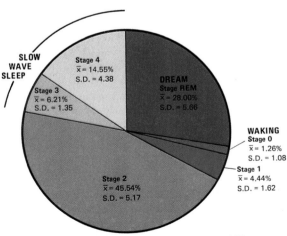

Figure 7-2
Normal composition
of sleep in a
young adult

PERCENTAGE OF SLEEP TIME FOR 20 - 29 YEAR-OLD MALES.
From R.L. Williams, I. Karacan and C.J. Hursch.
EEG of Human Sleep.
John Wiley & Sons, New York, 1974.

40

What If I Don't Sleep?

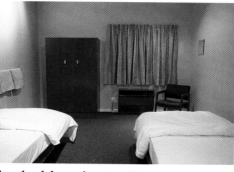

You do not need to worry about being able to sleep while in the laboratory. Patients are often concerned that they will be unable to sleep while wearing enough wiring to make them feel like a Christmas tree. Only rarely is a patient's sleep sufficiently disturbed by the lab environment to warrant an additional study. Most patients are surprised, even shocked, to find they have experienced a perfectly good night's sleep. In fact, people with chronic insomnia tend to sleep better on their first lab night than they do in their own homes.

Figure 7-3
A room in
a sleep lab

Will You Know What I Am Dreaming?

No. Although we are able to tell when you are in REM sleep (REM sleep is the time when most dreams occur), we cannot determine the content of your dreams.

Is It Painful?

No. There is usually no pain experienced during these procedures.

Why Do Some People Stay for Tests During the Day?

If sleepiness during the day appears to be an important issue, it is useful to conduct a multiple sleep latency test (MSLT) or a maintenance of wakefulness test (MWT). The patient stays in the lab on the day after their overnight study. Every two hours, the patient goes to bed and attempts to sleep or stay awake (depending on the instruction or test being performed). Since all electrodes are still in place from the previous night, we can tell how long it takes for the patient to fall asleep and what stages of sleep are attained. A patient who falls asleep in less than five minutes on most naps has a predisposition for irresistible daytime sleepiness, which may relate to the quality and quantity of sleep the night before. If REM sleep is noted during these daytime naps, in addition to irresistible sleepiness, then narcolepsy is suspected. If one cannot stay awake for approximately 13 minutes (on average) in the alertness test, then one's driving, for example, may be impaired.

Other Devices to Measure Insomnia

An *actigraph* detects body movements. It is worn on the wrist like an oversized watch. The actigraph helps us estimate total sleep time and, to a certain extent, sleep architecture and relative activity through the day.

An *Espie Device* measures the time of sleep onset. It has a

41

gentle spring-loaded mechanism which is compressed in the palm of the hand. The spring is released when the patient falls asleep.

The *Electrostatic Bed* is similar to the wrist actigraph in that it uses movement to estimate sleep. It is somewhat more accurate as it uses whole-body movements instead of single-limb movement. Of course, it does not provide any measure of activity outside of the bed.

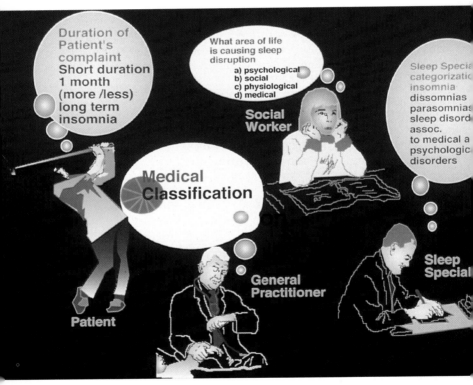

Figure 8-1
There are different ways of thinking about insomnia

What Are the Causes of Insomnia?

I n trying to help you establish why you are having bad sleep, and how you yourself can overcome it, we must remember that self-diagnosis and self-treatment are not always sufficient without medical aid; however, for many people sleep disruption is the result of an individual behavior pattern. The person who knows your behavior pattern best is you. Only by carefully examining your behavior is it likely that you or a doctor will be able to determine the cause of your insomnia. By examining the different ways in which doctors, psychologists, and others look at the causes of insomnia (Figure 8-1), we hope to provide clues to the various ways in which you might be disrupting your own sleep. In all of these categorizations the issues of quantity of sleep and quality of sleep apply.

Which Part of the Night Is Disrupted? (Figure 8-2)

This is an important way to classify insomnia. Insomniacs can be assorted into four categories:

People who have difficulty falling asleep. An example might be someone who is particularly worried about a business deal going sour, or adolescent children coming home late. However, once asleep, she has no difficulty in remaining asleep. If there are any consequences the next day, it is largely because of a shortened sleep duration.

People who wake up early in the morning and then remain awake. This occurs for a variety of reasons. It might simply be because of jet lag that the body clock and the environmental time are out of sync. It may be because of some emotional distress. Particularly in individuals suffering from depression, there may be early morning awakening with difficulty in returning to sleep.

People Who Have Difficulty Staying Asleep. A pain-related problem, such as rheumatoid arthritis, can be the cause. A pregnant woman, or a man with an enlarged prostate, may have to urinate repeatedly during the night. Awakenings in the middle of the night may be a consequence of withdrawal from medication, or of taking alcohol in the evening. Similarly, a patient taking L-dopa, an anti-Parkinsonian medication, might find that the drug has worn off causing a disruption of sleep.

43

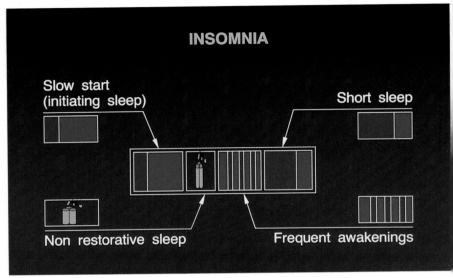

INSOMNIA

Slow start
(initiating sleep)

Short sleep

Non restorative sleep

Frequent awakenings

Figure 8-2
Another way of categorizing the type of insomnia you may have

People Who Have "Normal" Sleep but Poor Daytime Alertness and Concentration. Two common reasons are sleep apnea which is a breathing disorder during sleep, and nocturnal myoclonus, commonly known as restless legs syndrome. These people may think they are having a good sleep but they are mistaken (Figure 8-1).

What Area of Life is Causing Sleep Disruption?

This is the second categorization. Here again, there are four major divisions to consider, often found in combination with one another.

Psychological Problems: Insomnia may result from anxiety, depression, or other minor worry or major psychological stress (Figure 8-3). Many people who suffer from psychological or psychiatric disease have major sleep disruption. A patient with the eating disorder anorexia nervosa may have poor sleep including frequent sleep disruption because of low body mass and problems in controlling body temperature as well as psychological causes.

Traumatic experiences such as a major motor vehicle accident, assault, or rape may contribute to what psychiatrists call post-traumatic stress disorder. Many such individuals will have flashback experiences and may have interrupted sleep as well as nightmares.

Social Problems: Included in this category are work situations and marital discord, particularly if it leads to sexual

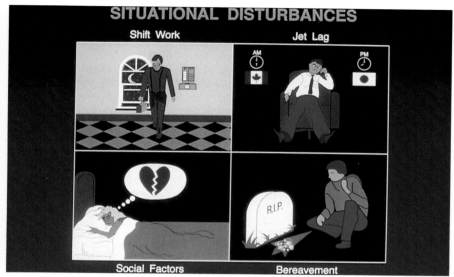

SITUATIONAL DISTURBANCES

Shift Work   Jet Lag

Social Factors   Bereavement

Figure 8-3
Life stresses can lead to insomnia

frustration. Tension within the relationship can frustrate communication and intimate sexual contact. This may lead to two individuals having little sleep, lying quietly in bed beside each other pretending to be asleep. As a consequence, they may be more irritable the next day because of shortened sleep, which leads to increased frustration and irritability — a vicious cycle.

Physiological Factors: In a very few individuals, it may be simply that their "sleep system" is not working as usual for unknown reasons. For these people long-term use of hypnotic medication is, in our view, appropriate. Other physiological causes of poor sleep quality are jet lag and those described in chapter 4.

Medical Factors: There is a huge array of reasons why a person might have difficulty falling asleep. An example is the individual with cancer who may worry about treatment, life expectancy, side effects of drugs, and may suffer the disruption of the disease process itself, causing poor sleep quality. As another example, a person with kidney failure may have increased daytime sleepiness because of the toxic material building up in the bloodstream that is not eliminated by the kidneys. An individual on dialysis may have variously too much or too little fluid causing marked sleep disruption. Patients may be on a variety of medications and these may directly affect their sleep. In a medical condition there may be factors that promote sleep or sleepiness, possibly at the wrong times of the day, and others that cause disruption of sleep. The balance of these effects will have a net effect in causing sleep disruption.

Medical Classification of Insomnia

A condition such as chest pain, which might suggest a heart attack, is one of the most frequently evaluated medical symptoms; however only one in 14 individuals with chest pain will visit his physician. For people with insomnia, only one in 256 will consult a physician. You can imagine that even the family physician is likely seeing a very select group of insomniacs. Another reason that the problem of insomnia is undertreated is that many see their doctor and complain of other things as well and the insomnia is somewhat dismissed. When you have read the consequences of insomnia (chapter 5) you will see why we do not think that insomnia should be ignored. Not only daytime performance, but also health and longevity are influenced by insomnia.

ETIOLOGY OF INSOMNIA

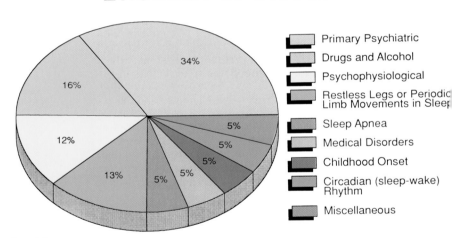

Figure 8-4

The pie diagram in Figure 8-4 shows a fairly typical distribution of complaints of patients with insomnia presenting at a sleep clinic. The most common diagnosis is a psychological or psychiatric cause which accounts for one-third of all insomniacs seen in a specialized clinic. This would include patients with anxiety and depression. One-sixth have drug or alcohol related problems which cause their sleep disruption.

A common but poorly understood condition is nocturnal myoclonus which is also known as periodic limb movement disorder (chapter 16). It accounts for one in eight insomniacs seen in a sleep clinic.

Psychophysiological insomnia accounts for approximately 1

percent of insomniacs. Usually these people have been light sleepers through most of their lives. It occurs more often in women than in men and is often related to a time in which they learned to have poor sleep. As an example, a trauma such as the death of a grandmother, may cause disrupted sleep during the bereavement. The issues of the loss are gradually resolved, but the problem of sleep disruption continues. Another example might be the university student studying for and worrying about forthcoming exams. The worry may be associated with disrupted sleep. The exams may come and go, the student may succeed in the examinations, but the insomnia may persist.

There is a group of medical conditions that have an associated sleep disruption. In some cases these medical conditions are not clearly diagnosed or the sleep disruption may be the first clue to the condition. Nocturnal asthma is one example. Particularly in children, this may present itself simply as a nighttime cough, and may not be recognized as asthma. One-third of adult asthmatics, have symptoms only at night. Although the phenomenon was described hundreds of years ago, only recently have doctors begun to deal with it. Ironically, there are numerous drugs used for nocturnal asthma which may disrupt sleep. The balance between treatment of the underlying condition and the side effects of the drugs must be taken into account. Invariably, it is the treatment of the underlying condition which relieves the problems and outweighs any specific problems caused by the treatment. A simple strategy, such as ensuring that the bedding is not susceptible to house-dust mite infestation, is important and can be easily achieved (Appendix).

A final group, including patients with dramatic sleep hygiene problems — for example, the pre-bedtime jogger or the person who consumes excessive amounts of coffee — may have insomnia. Many of the other conditions causing insomnia have poor sleep hygiene as an added component.

Sleep Specialist Categorization of Insomnia (Figure 8-1)

Specialists have devised a classification and categorization of sleep disorders. Among each of these categories, there are specific disorders in which insomnia is a major component. Among the intrinsic sleep disorders are 12 different conditions, five of which typically exhibit insomnia: psychophysiological insomnia; periodic limb movement disorder; restless legs syndrome; idiopathic insomnia; and sleep state misperception. An example of sleep state misperception was a man who, having been hit on the head by a forklift truck at Heathrow Airport, claimed not to sleep at all. On his third night in the sleep laboratory he slept for a couple of hours. Subsequently, he went

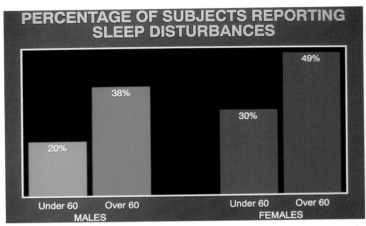

PERCENTAGE OF SUBJECTS REPORTING
SLEEP DISTURBANCES

49%

38%

30%

20%

Under 60   Over 60   Under 60   Over 60
MALES   FEMALES

Figure 8-5

to a second laboratory and was featured on the BBC as the only man in the world who did not sleep at all. His claims about his sleep were dramatically wrong.

On the other hand, idiopathic insomnia implies that the cause is unknown. Here there is a clear insomnia, usually combined with poor daytime functioning. It often starts in early childhood if not at birth. There is no overt medical or psychiatric disorder, nor any other specific sleep disorder. In idiopathic insomnia an individual often sleeps well on the first night in the sleep clinic but not as well subsequently — the reverse of what would occur for most people. For these rare individuals, long-term hypnotic medication may be particularly effective.

There are 13 extrinsic sleep disorders, eight of which are associated with difficulty either in initiating or maintaining sleep. These include inadequate sleep hygiene (the subject of another chapter); environmental sleep disorder; altitude insomnia; adjustment sleep disorder; sleep-onset association disorder; food allergy insomnia; hypnotic dependent sleep disorder; stimulant dependent sleep disorder; and alcohol dependent sleep disorder. The latter three are discussed in chapters 13 and 14.

Food allergy insomnia is more common in young children. Sensitivity to cow's milk may cause insomnia, which is resolved when milk is eliminated from the diet.

Even when a careful history and detailed notes about sleep and sleep problems are taken, only 50 percent of insomniacs receive a correct diagnosis and many will require a sleep study.

If the cause of the insomnia is clear, the treatment often becomes much easier. You may feel that one important classification not mentioned above is the duration of insomnia (Figure 8-1). This too will affect treatment. As people get older they have more sleep complaints (Figure 8-5).

CHAPTER NINE

Is Stress a Cause of your Insomnia?

he next few chapters cover five of the most common causes of insomnia that are not usually well assessed. We use a questionnaire to evaluate whether a particular problem applies to you. It would be surprising if all subjects were applicable to you and equally surprising if none applied. They account for more than 75 percent of all causes of insomnia. Therefore it is important you evaluate yourself in all four chapters.

The questionnaire offers broad coverage; most people suffering from a particular problem will be identified by it. The test is not infallible. The results of one test may incorrectly include a few without that problem. You should regard these questionnaires as guides and not as a final answer or diagnosis. If you score positively on any questionnaire, it is important that you speak to your family doctor about the issue. In some cases, your doctor may refer you to a medical specialist or to a sleep clinic to get you the right sort of help.

In this chapter we cover stress. The questionnaire tries to determine whether stress is a major feature in your life. It does not indicate whether stress is the cause of your insomnia.

Answer all questions by marking your response in the book. You will be able to refer to it later and, together with other recorded information, it will form a manual about your sleep. Repeating the questionnaire at a later stage will lend insight into how you have changed and the impact of the change on your sleep. When you repeat the questionnaire you should not be influenced by your "first time" responses.

Stress is a fact of every day life. It can be defined as any event which causes a significant emotional response. Even festive occasions such as weddings, promotions, or vacations can cause stress reactions, not only through participation in the event but also in the preparation. More obvious sources of stress are unhappy events: bereavement, divorce, loss of job. In such major life changes, the source of the emotional response is much more easily identified. Stress can also be triggered by rather trivial matters: an unironed shirt or a missed bus can create almost the same immediate emotional response.

There are two types of stress: *bad stress* or negative stress

which undermines your ability to operate at capacity, mentall
and physically; and *good stress* which improves performance –
the best example is a runner anticipating the starting gun. Hi
heart begins to race, breathing starts to increase, and menta
anxiety soars with the prospect of winning and the fear of losing
This is the type of stress that improves performance.

The type of stressors identified for the runner could b
considered negative responses in another situation, as in th
office or home. Stress then becomes a juggling act. Too littl
stress, both mental and physical, creates an unchallenged system
which cannot operate at its peak. Too much stress overloads th
faculties, leaving the most capable individual faltering. This i
displayed on the Yerkes-Dodson Curve (Figure 9-1).

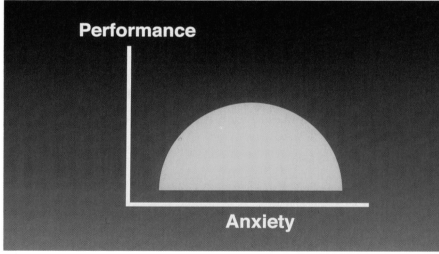

Figure 9-1
Both too little or
too much stress
lead to poor
performance

Stress is necessary for a healthy mind and body. You mus
exercise against resistance to achieve physical fitness. Exercisin
in thin air is not nearly as effective as exercising in water or wit
weights. Yet physical activity beyond your limits will give rise t
physical pain, weakness, and even physical damage. The same i
true of the human mind. The brain requires challenge in order t
maintain mental fitness. Too little challenge leaves us bored an
disinterested. Too many challenges render the mind unable t
cope with incoming messages. The mind that is challenged dail
yet has time for rest and orderly management of thos
challenges, is the mind of a mentally fit individual.

Stress is a subjective experience. Physical and menta
challenges that are a burden to one person may be trivial or eve
entertaining to another. How you perceive the challeng
determines how it will affect you. Effective stress managemen

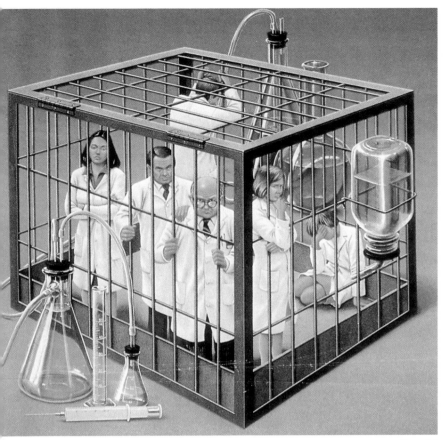

volves your identifying negative stressors and either removing
hem from your daily life or building up a resistance to them. By
ncreasing your tolerance or endurance in one area, you can
ctually increase resilience in other, seemingly unrelated areas.
ncreasing your physical fitness can often relieve the anxiety felt
efore delivering a public speech. Learning how to control an
motional reaction toward a given situation may improve your
hysical performance as in the case of the sprinter crouched in
nticipation of the starter's pistol.

Stress is a common phenomenon. One form of stress we
ear a lot about is referred to as "burnout" (Figure 9-2).

Try to answer the following questions with candor.

IDENTIFY YOUR STRESSORS

There are many day to day conditions which we find
tressful. The questions below ask you about your feelings and
houghts during the past month. In each case, you are asked to
ndicate how often you felt or thought a certain way. Although

some of the questions are similar, there are differences betwe[en]
them and you should treat each one as a separate question. T[he]
best approach is to answer each question fairly quickly. That [is]
don't try to count up the number of times you felt a particu[lar]
way, but rather indicate the alternative that seems a *reasona[ble]*
estimate. Please note your answer in the space provided at t[he]
end of each question. There are no *correct* answers; the aim is [to]
discover *your* thoughts and feelings.

For each question, please choose *only one* answer from t[he]
following alternatives:

0=never   1=almost never   2=sometimes   3=fairly often   4=very oft[en]

1. In the last month, how often have you been upset
    because of something that happened unexpectedly? _____

2. In the last month, how often have you felt that you
    were unable to control the important things in
    your life?   _____

3. In the last month, how often have you felt nervous
    and "stressed"?   _____

4. In the last month, how often have you dealt
    successfully with irritating life hassles?   _____

5.* In the last month, how often have you felt that you
    were effectively coping with important changes
    that were occurring in your life?   _____

6.* In the last month, how often have you felt confident
    about your ability to handle your personal problems?_____

7.* In the last month, how often have you felt that
    things were going your way?   _____

8. In the last month, how often have you found that
    you could not cope with all the things that you
    had to do?   _____

9.* In the last month, how often have you been able
    to control irritations in your life?   _____

10.* In the last month, how often have you felt that
    you were on top of things?   _____

1. In the last month, how often have you been
   angered because of things that were outside
   your control?   _____

2. In the last month, how often have you found
   yourself thinking about things that you
   have to accomplish?   _____

3.* In the last month, how often have you been
   able to control the way you spend your time?   _____

4. In the last month, how often have you felt
   difficulties were piling up so high that you
   could not overcome them?   _____

                                         Total   _____

Having completed the scale, please go back and alter your
answers opposite the asterisks (*) as follows: if you scored a 0,
put a 4; if a 1, put a 3; a 2, do not alter; if 3, put a 1; if a 4, put a 0.
Now total your score. The maximum score is 56. A score above
5 indicates that stress may be playing a major part in the
development of your insomnia.

There are three specific areas of your life where proper
management can increase resistance to negative stress:

Physical Management

Exercise tones your muscles, improves your cardiovascular
system, relaxes your body, and even changes your brain
chemistry for a healthier state of mind. What you eat is just as
important. Excessive cholesterol, fat, sugar, salt, alcohol, and
nicotine have negative effects on your ability to deal with stress.
Today's society is characterized by decreased physical activity
and increased availability of every type of food one can imagine.
The result is a population of overweight, physically unfit
individuals remarkably unable to fend off physical challenge. It
only makes sense that these physical shortcomings will affect
your state of mind. Feeling you no longer have adequate physical
stamina, you may begin to depend on a variety of aids to help you
through your daily routine. Caffeine, nicotine, sugar, cola, and
chocolate are used to simulate the sensation of physical and
mental fitness. Lack of physical activity, poor eating habits, and
the use of stimulants during the day give rise to a pattern of poor
sleep. A vicious cycle begins to unfold!

Personal Management

Social Support: Make time for friends. A strong soci support system improves physical and mental well-being an even lengthens life. Kindling new friendships and nurturing re-establishing old ones will decrease stress. Nothing can tak your mind off your troubles better than good times with goc friends.

Sense of Humor: Although we don't fully understand wh laughter has positive effects on your physical and ment well-being. Try to enjoy the humor in others while leaving roor to appreciate the humor within yourself.

Hobbies: It is important to engage in activities that remov you from everyday stress while allowing a sense accomplishment. Whether it is home improvements, golfing, knitting, an activity unrelated to your daily work provides yc with an important distraction from stress. However, beware hobbies that induce stress. If your golf game becomes over competitive, it may create as much stress as your work. Then is time to review your priorities. Few things induce sleep bett than focusing on the achievements or goals of a hobby whi lying peacefully with your eyes closed.

Personal Reward: If you have worked hard and have th means to buy that car, boat, dress, or piano of your dreams, the go for it! Allow the source of your stress to also be the source your reward.

Professional Management

Time Off and Holidays: Do not become a prisoner of you work. Lunch breaks, exercise breaks, adequate time at hom and holidays are all essential to your mental health. Eating sandwich while continuing with your work *does not* constitute lunch break. Taking along both your family and a bulgin briefcase does not constitute a holiday for them or you. You mu learn to escape from your work completely. This is not alway easy, but with effort and some reorganization you can improv matters. Remember, the hardest workers are not always th smartest or the most productive. They often spend more tim spinning their wheels as a result of relentless stress.

Time Management: Here are several principles fc effective time management: do the big jobs first; set prioritie shut your door (until you feel caught-up); schedule your da realistically.

Career Goals: Decide where you want your career to g and then work toward that goal. Be realistic. Progress alway involves work, time, and strategy. Strategy without work endless work without strategy leaves you stagnating. Decide a what level your own personal qualifications and standards allow you to perform best.

Career Changes: Unhappy with your work? Make changes. You can change your job or you can change elements of your existing job. Don't be afraid to make your feelings known to your employer and your family.

The following mnemonic to "**DOWN STRESS**" provides ten tips for coping with stress and burnout:

Don't delay relaxation. Use some relaxation technique daily.

Organize time well and delegate tasks. Leave spare time for emergencies.

Work off stress by doing some physical activity.

Negotiate and recognize what cannot be changed.

Sleep is a key to getting over stress.

Tiredness can go unrecognized, especially when under pressure.

Restrict use of alcohol, nicotine, coffee, and medications such as tranquilizers.

Establish regular, agreeable relaxations, such as walking the dog.

Say "no" now. This will prevent pressure in the future.

Sickness should not be ignored or "worked through".

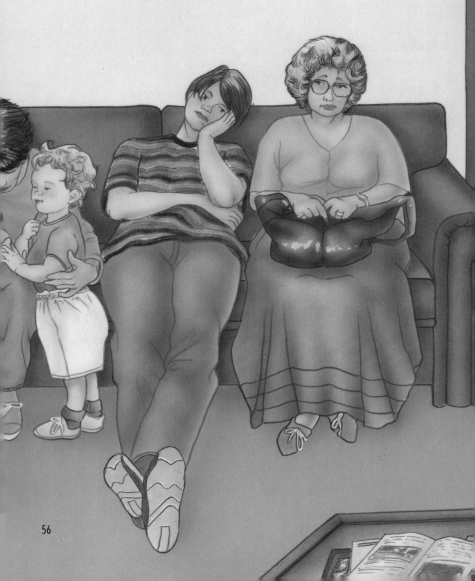

Figure 10-1
Anxiety can alter sleep.
Worry about medical matters,
for example, as with
these people waiting in a
doctor's office, may be the
trigger leading to poor sleep
and other problems

Do You Have Anxiety?

Anxiety is a common condition typified by a feeling of dread, accompanied by physical signs which indicate an overactive autonomic nervous system.

The physical signs (A to I) and psychological symptoms (A to I) of anxiety are listed in Tables 10-1 and 10-2.

Table 10-1: Physical Signs

Autonomic hyperactivity:
   tachycardia and palpitations; urinary frequency; diarrhea;
   dry mouth; sweating; flushing and pallor; cold hands
Backache
Catchy breathing and hyperventilation
Difficulty swallowing
Edginess and startled response
Fatiguability
Going numb - paresthesia
Headache
Inflexible muscles - muscle tension

Table 10-2: Psychological Symptoms

Anxious tension — angst
Butterflies in the stomach
Concentration difficulties
Decreased libido
Extreme worry
Feelings of dread
"Going crazy" sensation
Hypervigilance
Insomnia

Approximately one in ten people at some time suffers from anxiety. It is therefore a common cause of insomnia. Anxiety is both common and normal, as well as being a psychological disorder. We are all familiar with the anxiety associated with

Table 10-3: Canadian Clinical Anxiety Scale

	0	1	2	3	4
Psychic tension	No feeling of being tense	Slight tension — not distressing	Slight tension — mildly distressing	Tense as in category "4", but fluctuates during the day	Marked feeling of being "on edge", "keyed up", or "nervous" throughout wakefulness
Ability to relax	No subjective muscular tension	Slight tension — does not cause distress — can include mild headache	Definite muscular tension causing some distress	As in category "4", but only in some muscle groups — fluctuates during the day	Severe tension through most muscles linked with pain, stiffness, lack of control over movements occurs throughout the day. Cannot relax at will
Startle response	Similar to normal population	Slightly jumpy — but not distressing	Unexpected noise causes definite, but not severe, distress	Unexpected noise causes severe physical or mental distress	Unexpected noise or fright leads to sweating, heart racing, muscle activity, in addition to subjective anxiety — a feeling of "jumping out of your skin"
Worrying	Worrying is normal in relation to realistic circumstances (e.g., real financial crisis should be worried about)	You worry more than is necessary about minor matters — no significant distress	Painful thoughts out of proportion with your situation — but you can dismiss them	As in category "4", but fluctuation in intensity — may stop periodically during the day	Continuous preoccupation with painful thoughts which are out of proportion and cannot be stopped
Apprehension	Anticipation of something bad	Slight apprehension not causing much distress	Some unsubstantiated apprehension of disaster causing definite distress	As in category "4", but not more than once a day	Feeling close to the brink of some disaster may occur all day or repeatedly across the day
Restlessness	None	Slight but not causing distress	Needing to be "on the move". Causing mild distress	As in category "4", but can keep still for one hour at a time	Unable to keep still for a few minutes — restless pacing and other purposeless activity

asks that need to be completed. Concern about taking a driving
test or other new or unknown experience may cause some sense
of worry. When anxiety leads to poor sleep a cycle may develop
wherein the worry over sleep in itself prevents sleep; it becomes a
self-fulfilling prophecy. In some cases this develops into a more
overwhelming situation.

There are many medical causes of anxiety, including low
blood sugar, fever, chronic infections, thyroid disease, mitral
valve prolapse, and angina. Hyperventilation associated with
anxiety can worsen anxiety symptoms. Breathing into a paper
bag will help.

Scoring Your Anxiety

On the table on page 58, please tick-off the box on each row
which best applies to you. This scale is an instrument to assess
your present state of anxiety. Your response should relate to how
you feel at the present time. Once completed, add up your score
using the numbers at the top of each column. The following is a
guide to your level of anxiety: Normal, less than 4; Mild, 5-10;
Moderate, 11-16; Severe, 17-24.

Coping With Anxiety

One of the best ways to cope with anxiety is to list the issues
that provoke it. Write each item on a single card or sheet of
paper, then group the items into various *categories*. You may
have concerns about the home, (the plumbing needs repairing or
bills need paying); concerns at work, (a particular deadline has to
be met or a confrontation with a boss is looming). You may also
be facing interpersonal issues or difficult financial matters.

Having made these categories you should decide which
ones to tackle the *next day*, and which ones might be dealt with
the *next week*. Note this on the cards. In this way you will be able
to divide and conquer the problems. At bedtime you will have
fewer issues floating around in your head and they will not
overwhelm you. There is no substitute for acting to resolve the
problems underlying your anxiety. By reducing the number of
conflicts or problems, you will be less anxious in the future. The
other advantage of noting the sources of anxiety is elimination of
the worry about forgetting the important issues you have to deal
with. Furthermore, if something new comes into your mind at
that time, you will know that there will be a regular time, perhaps
after dinner each day, when you will be able to think about this
and note it on your cards. Also note issues resolved and keep a
"dealt with" pile.

This is one aspect of one behavioral strategy which is useful for
anxiety, but it is helpful also in other causes of insomnia. Further
information about behavioral strategies is provided in chapter 20.

59

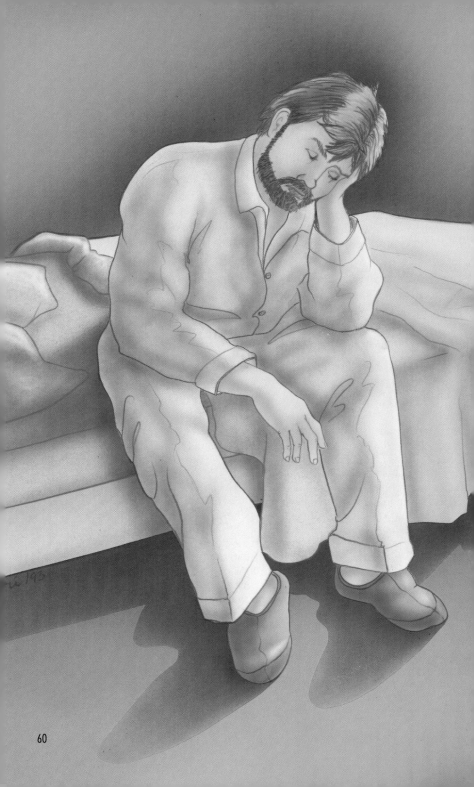

CHAPTER ELEVEN

Is Depression a Cause of your Insomnia?

F eeling sad or happy is part of normal experience. A lasting feeling of extremely low mood, either triggered by an external event or arising from within, may occur. These changes have a specific character and constitute an illness. In some cases there may be a family history of depression. There is often a clear positive response to appropriate treatment. In more than 90 percent of patients with depression there is a change in sleep and, in many, there are increased awakenings during the night; less deep sleep in the first sleep cycle; and REM sleep occurring earlier in the night. Insomnia is a very common feature. The following scale allows you to assess whether you are experiencing depression. Carry out the exercise as honestly as you can giving the response that applies closest to you.

CES-D SCALE

Below is a list of the ways you might have felt or behaved. Please indicate how often you have felt this way *during the past week*.

- Rarely or none of the time (Less than 1 day)
- Some or a little of the time (1 - 2 days)
- Occasionally or a moderate amount of time (3 - 4 days)
- Most or all of the time (5 - 7 days)

	Rarely/ None	Some/ A Little	Occasionally/ Moderately	Most/ All
I was bothered by things that usually don't bother me.	0	1	2	3
I did not feel like eating; my appetite was poor.	0	1	2	3
I felt that I could not shake off the blues even with help from my family and friends.	0	1	2	3
I felt that I was just as good as other people.	3	2	1	0

	Rarely/ None	Some/ A Little	Occasionally/ Moderately	Most/ All
5. I had trouble keeping my mind on what I was doing.	0	1	2	3
6. I felt depressed.	0	1	2	3
7. I felt that everything I did was an effort.	0	1	2	3
8. I felt hopeful about the future.	3	2	1	0
9. I thought my life had been a failure.	0	1	2	3
10. I felt fearful.	0	1	2	3
11. My sleep was restless.	0	1	2	3
12. I was happy.	3	2	1	0
13. I talked less than usual.	0	1	2	3
14. I felt lonely.	0	1	2	3
15. People were unfriendly.	0	1	2	3
16. I enjoyed life.	3	2	1	0
17. I had crying spells.	0	1	2	3
18. I felt sad.	0	1	2	3
19. I felt that people disliked me.	0	1	2	3
20. I could not get going.	0	1	2	3

Now add up your total score. If you have scored more than 17 on the above questionnaire, you should consult your family doctor. This book is aimed at helping you to sleep (and it is true that sleep disruption can cause depression), but it does not purport to give advice about the treatment of specific conditions such as depression or alcohol dependence.

Recall that early morning awakening was described as being characteristic of depression. There are few other conditions in which this pattern is seen. However, it is most common for depressed people to have difficulty in falling asleep, (i.e., more common than having early morning awakening). Difficulty falling asleep is also triggered by many other causes and so is less specific to depression.

CHAPTER TWELVE

Do You Have
Bad Sleep Hygiene?

ood sleep hygiene is 80 percent common sense and 20 percent understanding something about sleep. At this point you should have completed a sleep diary and recorded your daytime activities in relation to your sleep. You will have gathered that there is an interaction between daytime activities and nighttime sleep. You will have learned about the effects of exercise on sleep and of regular behavior patterns in relation to sleep. For example, a regular snack at bedtime will facilitate sleep, whereas an occasional snack might have more sleep-disruptive effects.

The purpose of this chapter is to document to what extent you follow simple sleep hygiene rules. You might feel that they are excessively strict and severe. There are many people who do not adhere to these rules who have good quality sleep. If *your* sleep is disrupted it may be that the breaking of some of these rules has a marked impact on *you*. The impact of a particular behavior differs in different people. For example, the effect of smoking on a person with asthma is different than that on a person who does not have asthma. The effect of alcohol on sleep is different in a young person as compared to an older person. Although some people may have certain behaviors which do not disrupt their sleep, it may be that those very same behaviors will disrupt *your* sleep. We therefore recommend that you improve as many behaviors as possible.

On the **Sleep Hygiene Chart**, you are asked to address each item and respond with your initial assessment. For example, the chart will remind you not to take daytime naps. If you do take occasional naps then you do not score well in this hygiene behavior. Not every rule applies to every person. For some individuals, a regular nap actually promotes nighttime sleep; but for most the reverse is true.

This chart affords a current assessment of your strengths and weaknesses in relation to sleep hygiene. It is not our role to dictate your lifestyle. If you believe that a couple of cups of coffee are part of the pleasure of daily living then you should take them early in the day, rather than after the evening meal. Decaffeinated coffee should be your choice. Some sleep hygiene-related effects

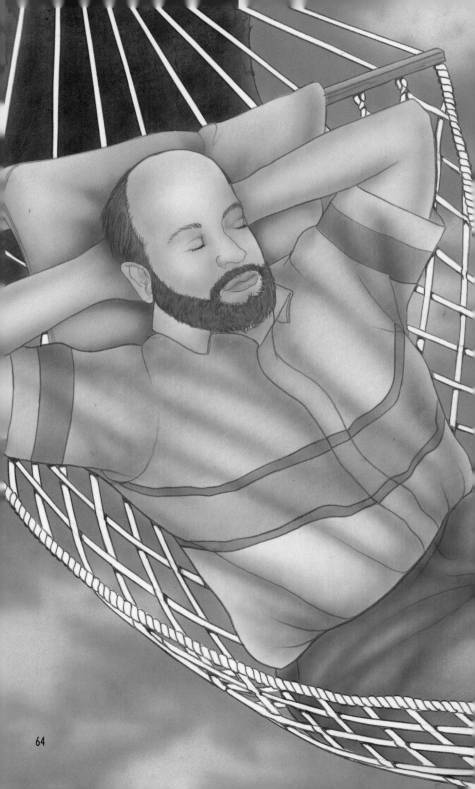

are beyond your control, such as noise. If you live adjacent to a highway, sound screening may be important. However, if a small child is waking you up, then dealing with the child's problem is an important step.

SLEEP HYGIENE CHART

			Good Hygiene	
1.	Do you wake at the same time each day?		Yes	No
2.	Do you exercise each day?		Yes	No
3.	Do you exercise close to bedtime?	Yes	No	
4.	Do you have much caffeine in a day?	Yes	No	
5.	Do you have any caffeine after 4:00 p.m.?	Yes	No	
6.	Do you set aside time daily to deal with stress, e.g., list next day's tasks?		Yes	No
7.	Do you smoke?	Yes	No	
8.	Do you smoke after 8:00 p.m.?	Yes	No	
9.	Do you have much to eat after 8:30 p.m.?	Yes	No	
10.	Do you consume much fluid after 8:30 p.m.?	Yes	No	
11.	Do you drink alcohol after 9:00 p.m.?	Yes	No	
12.	Do you have time to unwind before bedtime?		Yes	No
13.	Do you have regular behaviors before bedtime, e.g., light snack?		Yes	No
14.	Do you have a hot shower or bath before bed?		Yes	No
15.	Do you go to bed when drowsy?		Yes	No
16.	Do you occasionally nap in the day?	Yes	No	
17.	Have you discussed with your doctor any outstanding medical issues which may affect your sleep?		Yes	No
18.	Do you take non-prescription drugs?	Yes	No	
19.	Is your bed comfortable?		Yes	No
20.	Have you considered whether your bed partner is negatively affecting your sleep?		Yes	No
21.	Is sexual tension preventing you from falling asleep?	Yes	No	
22.	Do you engage in any stimulating activity before sleep, e.g., watching TV, sexual intercourse (for some), arguments?	Yes	No	
23.	Is your bedroom secure?		Yes	No
24.	Is your bedroom quiet and cool?		Yes	No
25.	Is your bedroom dark?		Yes	No

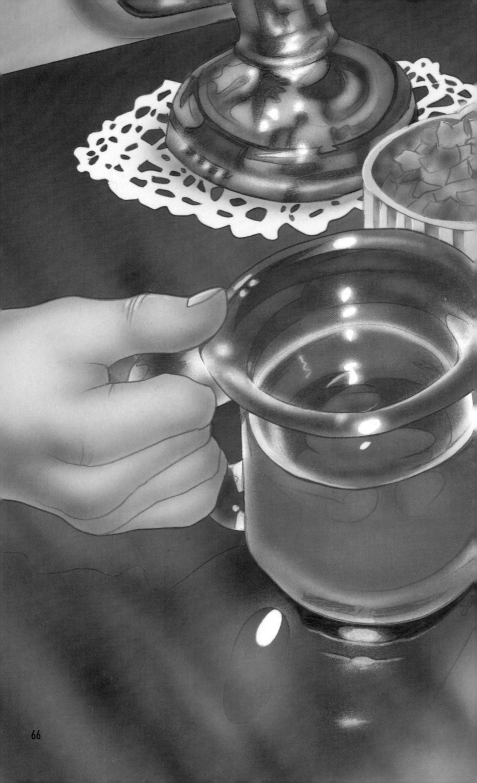

CHAPTER THIRTEEN

Is your Insomnia Related to Alcohol Consumption?

The consequences of life itself, our environment, our personalities, and the misuse and abuse of substances make us victims of sleep disturbances. About 77 percent of men and 60 percent of women in North America drink alcohol. The United States has the second highest rate of problem drinkers in the world. Approximately 7 percent of the adult population have alcohol problems. Abuse of alcohol is increasing in females although it is two to five times more common in males.

A neurochemical balance exists between brain centers controlling emotions, the reticular activating system (which controls arousal), and the sleep system, all of which regulate the state of our consciousness. Alcohol disturbs this balance.

Alcohol depresses both our anxiety and our active waking system. Hence, many fall asleep faster with a drink. A "drugged" sleep may follow for the next few hours. Thereafter, the drinker awakens repeatedly during the last two to three hours of sleep. Alcohol may increase an awareness of dreams and dreaming time. If the dreams are unpleasant, returning to sleep might be difficult. Increased urinary frequency and headache may also disrupt sleep.

After repeated use of alcohol, sleep becomes more fragmented and a serious problem develops. The body, physically and mentally, has had no time to heal and recover. Sufferers of sleep apnea have a worsening of snoring and more breathing irregularities after alcohol consumption. Alcohol specifically reduces muscle tone in the upper airway, increasing the likelihood of airway collapse.

When alcohol is withdrawn, fragmentation of sleep occurs. Dreaming becomes excessive (as a rebound) and this pattern lasts for up to ten days, often with nightmares and anxious dreams. In extreme cases there may be restlessness, anxiety, and tremors in the morning.

These disturbances resolve after two weeks of abstinence, but a complete return to normal sleep may take up to two years. If sleep dissatisfaction was the cause of excessive alcohol use, then normal sleep may be achieved through a program to improve sleep quality.

Many acquire their drinking habits in young adulthood. With time, the brain's sensitivity to alcohol and alcohol withdrawal changes. Many people who previously considered alcohol a useful inducer of sleep subsequently find they have disrupted sleep despite their alcohol consumption. This may be because the body metabolizes alcohol during the sleep period and withdrawal goes on all night. In a young individual the sleep drive may be sufficient to overcome the withdrawal process, but as he gets older the sleep drive is less robust and he is awakened as the level of alcohol in his bloodstream drops. The same applies to very short-acting sleeping pills, for example Triazolam (Halcion). The effect may be to cause early morning awakening with a sense of anxiety and shakiness. An awareness of the problem is usually sufficient to change the behavior pattern; most people would prefer to have better quality sleep than to continue drinking. However, many people do not recognize that they have this alcohol problem or related problems. We have included two short questionnaires which may be useful to you. The first is the **CAGE**, acronymic for Cut-down, Annoyed, Guilty, and Eye-opener. Complete these four questions by circling "yes" or "no".

Have you ever felt you should cut down
your drinking?   Yes No

Have people annoyed you by criticizing
your drinking?   Yes No

Have you ever felt bad or guilty about
your drinking?   Yes No

Have you ever had a drink first thing in the
morning (an eye-opener) to steady
your nerves or to get rid of a hang-over?   Yes No

If you have circled one "Yes", alcohol may be a problem.

The second questionnaire is the **MAST** (Michigan Alcoholism Screening Test). The usefulness of this test depends on your honesty. Circle your answers.

1. Do you feel you are a normal drinker?   Yes No

2. Have you ever awakened in the morning
    after some drinking the night before and
    found that you could not remember
    a part of the evening before?   Yes No

3. Does your spouse (or parent) ever worry
   or complain about your drinking? Yes No

4. Can you stop drinking without a struggle
   after one or two drinks? Yes No

5. Do you ever feel bad about your drinking? Yes No

6. Do friends or relatives think you are
   a normal drinker? Yes No

7. Are you always able to stop drinking
   when you want to? Yes No

8. Have you ever attended a meeting
   of Alcoholics Anonymous (AA)
   because of your drinking? Yes No

9. Have you gotten into fights when drinking? Yes No

10. Has drinking ever created problems with
    you and your spouse? Yes No

11. Has your spouse (or other family member)
    ever gone to anyone for help about your
    drinking? Yes No

12. Have you ever lost friends or boyfriends/
    girlfriends because of your drinking? Yes No

13. Have you ever gotten into trouble at work
    because of drinking? Yes No

14. Have you ever lost a job because of drinking? Yes No

15. Have you ever neglected your obligations,
    your family, or your work for two or more
    days in a row because you were drinking? Yes No

16. Do you ever drink before noon? Yes No

17. Have you ever been told you have
    liver trouble? Cirrhosis? Yes No

18. Have you ever had delirium tremens (DTs),
    severe shaking, heard voices, or seen things
    that were not there after heavy drinking? Yes No

19. Have you ever gone to anyone for help about your drinking?   Yes No

20. Have you ever been in a hospital because of your drinking?   Yes No

21. Have you ever been a patient in a psychiatric hospital or on a psychiatric ward of a general hospital when drinking was part of your problem?   Yes No

22. Have you ever been seen at a psychiatric or mental health clinic, or gone to a doctor, social worker, or clergyman for help with an emotional problem in which drinking had played a part?   Yes No

23. Have you ever been arrested, even for a few hours, because of drunken behavior?   Yes No

24. Have you ever been arrested for drunk driving or driving after drinking?   Yes No

Scoring Information

Alcohol problems are not a single issue, therefore, subsections of this questionnaire are considered. Add up the number of positive responses to items 3, 5, and 15, and the number of negative responses to items 1, 4, 6, and 7. You should get a score between 0 and 7. The higher the score, the more evidence that you *worry about your alcohol problems.*

If you now add up the number of positive responses for items 9, 12, 13, 14, 18, 23, and 24, a score between 0 and 7 will indicate whether you have *legal, work and social problems* related to your alcohol consumption. Once again, the higher the score, the more likely that you have problems.

Adding up the positive responses for items 8, 19, 20, 21, and 22, gives a score between 0 and 5 which indicates how *likely* you are *to seek help* for alcohol related problems.

If you add up the positive responses for items 3, 10, and 11, you will get a score between 0 and 3, which indicates whether there are *marital and/or family difficulties* related to your alcohol consumption.

If you have found that you have more problems than you anticipated, you should discuss this matter in earnest with your family physician. You should arrange for some specific help in cutting down your alcohol consumption as it is likely that this has a bearing on your sleep-related problems.

CHAPTER FOURTEEN

Drug Causes of Insomnia

Drugs may have a detrimental effect on your sleeping system. Some drugs cause insomnia during sustained use, either by directly stimulating the central nervous system or by the development of tolerance to the drug. Other drugs cause insomnia upon withdrawal of the drug, including benzodiazepines, major tranquilizers, pain relievers, cocaine, and opiates.

Drugs used for medical illnesses, seemingly unrelated to the central nervous system, may cause insomnia. These include drugs used in the treatment of asthma, heart failure, hypertension, thyroid disease, cancer chemotherapy, coughs and colds, and arthritis. The first objective is to establish whether a drug you are taking causes insomnia. Next, you will want to know if there is an alternative. Some similar drugs for high blood pressure differ dramatically in how easily the drug gets into the brain and causes disrupted sleep.

The following are central nervous system stimulants: nicotine, caffeine, cocaine, marijuana, ephedrine, pseudoephedrine, phenyl-propanolamine, phenylephrine, salbutamol, spasmolytic (anti-asthma) medications, amphetamines, non-amphetamine stimulants.

Nicotine is the most commonly abused stimulant in the world. Quickly absorbed into the blood, it reaches the brain eight seconds after inhalation. It stimulates release of adrenaline which stimulates the heart and increases alertness. The harmful effects of cigarette smoking on the lungs are well known. Smokers sleep, on average, half an hour less per night than non-smokers. When anxious, many smokers increase their nicotine consumption compounding their sleep and anxiety problems.

Tea, coffee, and chocolate all contain **caffeine**. It is also included in some over-the-counter pain relievers. Tea contains a related chemical, theophylline, which is also a stimulant. Caffeine increases wakefulness, body temperature, and mental alertness. Table 14 shows the amounts of caffeine in different beverages. The strength of the brew is important. The sensitivity of the individual is also a major factor. After age 40, many people previously impervious to the effect of caffeine find they have to give up evening coffee to sleep well. Insomniacs who find they are sleepy in the day because of a bad night may prop themselves up with caffeine. Excessive caffeine may then interfere with sleep the following night. They will then need even more caffeine to feel alert the following day. We urge you to acquire a taste for decaffeinated brands of coffee, cola, and other products on the list which you consume regularly.

TABLE 14: COMMON SOURCES OF CAFFEINE

Product		Caffeine
Instant coffee	1 cup	66 mg
Coffee - percolated	"	110 mg
Coffee - drip brewed	"	146 mg
Decaffeinated coffee	"	2-5 mg
Tea - brewed 1 minute	"	25 mg
Tea - brewed 5 minutes	"	46 mg
Cocoa	"	13 mg
Jolt Cola	12 ounce can	120 mg
Coca-Cola	"	60 mg
Dr. Pepper	"	60 mg
Tab	"	49 mg
Pepsi Cola	"	43 mg
Chocolate bar	approx. 2 ounces	25 mg

Non-Prescription Stimulants

Vivadrin	200 mg
Caffedrine	200 mg
No Doz	100 mg
Pre-mens Forte	100 mg
Aqua-Ban (over-the-counter diuretic)	100 mg

Non-Prescription Medications

Excedrin	64 mg
Vanquish	32 mg
Anacin	32 mg
Emprin	32 mg
Midol	32 mg
Dristan	16 mg

Cocaine is a powerful drug made from the cocoa shrub and derivatives are used as an anaesthetic during surgery. It is abused for its pleasurable effects by an alarming number of people. It stimulates the heart and central nervous system producing a false sense of well-being and alertness.

Amphetamines (diet pills) are potent sleep inhibitors. They stimulate the heart and the awake system and suppress the appetite centers. Other stimulants such as ephedrine, pseudo-ephedrine, phenylephrine, and phenylpropanolamine have a similar effect, but are used more often in cough and cold preparations.

Anti-asthma medications such as Salbutamol stimulate the heart and brain and cause insomnia. Theophylline, aminophylline, and oxytriphylline also aggravate the insomnia. An asthmatic can therefore have insomnia from a difficulty breathing, from problems of getting enough oxygen to the brain, from the anxiety of such a situation, and from the numerous stimulant medications taken. Some asthmatics have symptoms only at night. This can make treatment more complicated.

Marijuana — nicknamed grass, pot, or weed — is a drug made from dried leaves and flowers of the hemp plant. It contains 400 chemicals. When smoked, it produces more than 2,000 chemicals which enter the body. It may cause drowsiness and sleepiness, but the sleep is fragmented and the user wakes up tired and depressed in the morning.

The withdrawal of **opiates** such as opium, morphine, heroin, and codeine will produce severe insomnia. Used in the 1800s as the most effective pain reliever, opium also stops coughs and diarrhea and relieves anxiety. It is a depressant of the central nervous system and induces sleep with vivid dreams. Addiction rapidly develops producing profound dependence. Codeine, a metabolite of opium, is present in combination with acetaminophen, e.g., Tylenol 1, 2, 3. Hydrocodone (a more potent form of codeine) is found in cough syrups with a DH suffix. Drug seekers continually invent strange and heartbreaking stories when requesting these drugs from physicians.

Many **hypnotics** (sleep inducing medications) such as certain benzodiazepines and barbiturates initially induce sleep (nonREM Stages I and II) and suppress deep and REM sleep. They decrease anxiety and reduce sleep restlessness and vividness of dreams. The body's stress hormones, (corticosteroids) are also reduced. With prolonged use, the body tries to compensate for this unnatural state and increases its production of the stress hormones and other chemicals.

After a few weeks of using these these drugs, especially barbiturates and chloral hydrate, the brain also adjusts to the sleep inducing chemicals, making them less effective. More and more medication is needed to produce the same amount of sleep. This is known as *tolerance* to the drug. The insomnia may become worse than it was before the sleeping medication was started. To make matters worse, when medications are stopped, a more severe form of insomnia, rebound or recoil insomnia, occurs. Sleep becomes increasingly poor. Severe anxiety, restlessness, tremors, and irrational depression occur over a period of a few days to weeks. The experience is so unpleasant that many are afraid to stop taking their sleeping medication. Abrupt withdrawal from high dosages of benzodiazepine medication can be dangerous and may cause seizures. One way to safely withdraw from benzodiazepines is to switch to a new class of sleeping medication known as cyclopyrrolones (e.g., zopiclone) and to stop taking them after four weeks. The improvement in sleep quality in doing this is shown in Figure 14-1. The advantages of this approach are numerous and include:

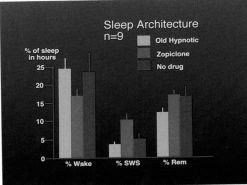

- Does not suppress deep sleep and may increase it, even after use of other hypnotics.
- Does not suppress REM sleep. Sleep structure is more normal than with benzodiazepine medications.
- Rebound on withdrawal of the drug is lessened or eliminated.
- The drug has more specific effects on sleep. Most benzodiazepines have muscle relaxant,

Figure 14-1
In this study, we recorded the sleep of a group of people taking benzodiazepine sleeping pills over a long period (> 4 months). They switched to zopiclone for one month, had their sleep recorded, and then stopped all sleep medications for one month. Some of the gains in sleep architecture after zopiclone are retained even after stopping the drug

as well as sleep effects. Generally, the more specific the action, as with cyclopyrrolones, the better.

Diuretics are commonly used in heart failure, high blood pressure, kidney failure, and conditions causing excess fluid in the body, especially in the elderly. They increase urination and this disrupts sleep at night especially when taken late in the day. Large amounts of electrolytes, such as potassium, are lost from the body with diuretics. A low potassium level may cause painful cramps which disrupt sleep.

Antidepressants and antipsychotic drugs used in psychiatric disturbances often alter sleep. Prozac (fluoxetine) particularly may disrupt sleep especially if taken late in the day and may require use of a sleeping medication at night.

Thyroid hormone replacement enhances the effect of the body's adrenaline in the blood. Dosage must be carefully determined, as a slightly excessive amount causes tremors, rapid heart rate, sweating, weight loss, irritability, and profound insomnia. A low level of the thyroid hormone has the opposite effect.

Beta blockers are **cardiovascular drugs** used in treating high blood pressure, angina, and heart diseases. They suppress REM sleep and can cause sleep disruptions, nightmares, and hallucinations. Switching from one beta blocker to another may have the same effect on the heart but resolve sleep problems.

Gastrointestinal irritants which cause stomach upset and pain include aspirin, alcohol, anti-inflammatories, antibiotics, and cancer treatment drugs. These agents may cause or aggravate a peptic ulcer of the stomach or duodenum. This can cause severe stomach or chest pain, vomiting, and even bleeding in the gastrointestinal tract. These are common causes of awakening at night

Medical Causes of Insomnia

he many medical causes of insomnia are listed below. Our purpose is not to overwhelm you, but to show how many conditions can contribute to poor sleep. They can be divided into two groups — those that produce pain and those that do not.

In the first group are **Headaches** including migraine; the cluster headache produced by stress; sleep apnea leading to headache; hypertension and aneurysm; neck pain and neck injury; and head injury: concussion or fractures. This group also includes **Ear, nose, and throat conditions** such as sinus infection, throat infection, croup and olitis; **Eye diseases** such as corneal abrasion, glaucoma (acute angle closure), flash burns or keratitis; and the **Cardiovascular diseases** of angina, myocardial infarction, aortic valvular disease, and pericarditis. **Gastrointestinal disorders** causing insomnia and characterized by pain include: hunger; hiatus hernia and hyperacidity; duodenal ulcer; gall stones and cholecystitis; appendicitis; obstructions, such as adhesions, volvulus (twisting of the bowel in on itself), and ischemia of the bowel in the elderly; and tumors. **Urogenital causes** are: infections of the urinary tract, prostatitis, and epididymitis; kidney and bladder stones; painful penile erections; and menstrual pains. **Musculoskeletal disorders** are: mechanical neck and back strains; arthritis and gout; fibrositis; and nocturnal leg cramps. **Cancers** of the pancreas, bone, and brain form the last group of pain-related causes.

Non-pain related causes of insomnia include **Nocturia** (urinating during the night) which is related to either aging, infection, recovery from acute glomerulonephritis, chronic renal failure, or bladder and prostatic tumors; **Endocrine diseases** which include diabetes with thirst, hypoglycemia due to insulin dosage and diabetic neuropathy, thyroid diseases, hyperthyroidism, and hypocalcemia causing muscular cramps and tetany; **Allergies**; **Asthma**; and **Drugs** (chapter 14).

Emotional and psychiatric causes of insomnia have been discussed in earlier chapters. The sleep-wake system receives messages from emotional centers, sensory organs receiving painful stimuli, and the higher brain centers. If you are busy

75

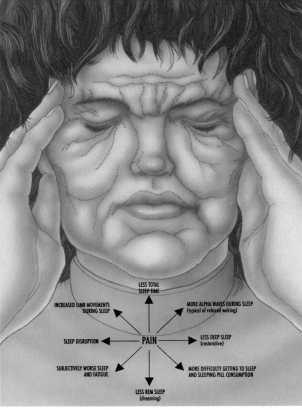

Figure 15-1
Pain disrupts sleep

during the day or asleep at night, your attention to pain may be low. However when lying awake in bed without any other focus, even minor pains may take on a major significance. When this awareness of pain prevents sleep, you may seek medical help for either the pain or the sleep disruption. The level of pain sensitivity varies at different stages of sleep (Figure 15-1).

Pain travels up the spinal cord from the pain receptors on the skin and organs via the thalamus which is like a central sensory processing unit in the brain. From there the message goes to other brain centers including the sleep-wake system.

In the head and neck all pain impulses travel via the trigeminal ganglion to the brain. This common path means that pains from many different causes are perceived as headache.

Headaches are a significant cause of sleep disruption. **Migraine** headaches are usually on one side of the head but may be on both. Initially a sharp pain is described around the eye or front of the head. This is followed by throbbing pain, flashes of light or a zig-zag visual image, and abdominal discomfort. Vomiting and nausea may accompany the headache. Bright lights may aggravate the pain so a dark room is sought. Various trigger factors include diet (vanilla, chocolate, bananas, cherries, alcohol), changes in atmospheric pressure (approaching storms) and emotional and physical stress such as menstruation. Sleep may help this pain. **Cluster** headaches occur mainly in males in their 20s and 30s and are about twice as common at night. The pain begins just above the eyebrow and spreads to that side of the head. It is associated with tearing, runny nose, redness of the eye, and sweating on one side of the head. These symptoms appear to occur immediately after REM sleep.

Interrupted breathing at night is seen mainly in

overweight older men sometimes resulting in sleep apnea. An accumulation of carbon dioxide and a fall of oxygen may ensue. This produces a throbbing morning headache which clears without treatment several hours after rising.

High blood pressure commonly produces tightness around the head. It is often worse in the mornings. Awakening during the night with a headache may be a complication of high blood pressure and should be taken as warning of a possible stroke. High blood pressure has been associated with sleep apnea and/or snoring. A rare but important cause of morning headache is that observed by a student GP when a few people from one apartment building came in to see him, all complaining of morning headaches. It seems that the building incinerator had broken down. One flap had been jammed open, allowing for the release of carbon monoxide, and all the people on the top floor of the building were being poisoned by carbon monoxide at night.

Ear, nose, and throat infections: The pain from these conditions, which is particularly marked at night, commonly causes insomnia. Lying down results in poor drainage of these areas which aggravates the problem. This is why many ear infections in children are most troublesome at night.

Eye pain: The symptoms of **Glaucoma** (acute angle closure) are extreme pain, redness, blurred vision, watery eye, and a dilated nonreactive pupil. Treatment must be sought within 12 to 48 hours after onset of the pain or blindness may result. The condition can be triggered by a dark environment or in sleep.

Cardiovascular causes: **Myocardial infarction** (heart attack) occurs mostly at rest especially in the latter part of the sleeping period (perhaps related to dream sleep) and in the early mornings (perhaps related to the process of awakening and getting out of bed). The pain is severe. Weakness, cold sweats, restlessness, nausea and vomiting, and apprehension may be present.

Gastrointestinal disorders: **Hunger** commonly causes awakening. Acidic fluid irritates the lining of an empty stomach. A snack before bedtime may aid sleep. **Heartburn** (acid reflux) commonly occurs with a hiatus hernia in which the stomach slides partially into the chest. This is worse in the night, lying down after a meal, or when in a squatting position. Often a person awakens out of a deep sleep with a sour acidic taste in the back of the mouth or with the sensation of choking. Antacids, diet, postural change, and, for many, weight reduction, are

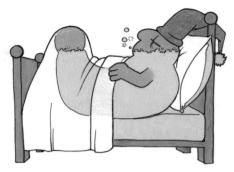

beneficial. Alcohol use aggravate the problem. Using a bed which allows a semi-sitting position can be quite helpful (Figure 15-2). **Ulcer** of the duodenum typically disrup sleep in the early hours of the morning with a burning pain in the stomach. This is relieved by food and antacids. Stress, hyperactivity diet, alcohol, and drugs are common precipitating causes.

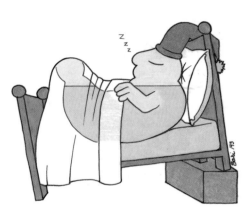

Urogenital problems: Bladder and kidney infections cause frequent painful urination which may awaken you from sleep. There is usually pain in the lower abdomen or back and fever. In some men there may be painful erections which occur during REM sleep and cause awakening.

Musculoskeletal disorders: Commonly, **neck and back pain** sufferers are restless at night and they often take pain relievers with a sedative (e.g., acetaminophen with

Figure 15-2
Raise the head
of the bed to
decrease reflux

codeine). This affects about 50 percent of the population at some time during their lives and 1 to 2 percent become chronically impaired with neck and back pain. **Fibromyalgia** is commonly associated with generalized musculoskeletal aches, morning stiffness, fatigue headaches, neck pain, and sleep disturbances. It occurs mainly in women. Correcting the sleep disorder with low doses of antidepressants or a cyclopyrrollone may be beneficial (chapter 21). **Carpal tunnel syndrome** is a common painful disorder of the wrist and hands felt usually at night. Numbness and a tingling sensation may precede the pain which may spread upward to the arm. Repetitive use of hands, injuries to the wrist arthritis, hypothyroid disease, pregnancy, and conditions causing fluid retention may cause the problem. Night splints or surgery may be therapeutic. **Arthritis** causes pain, swelling and stiffness of joints. Insomnia is a feature especially in the severe acute phase. **Gout** causes severe inflammation of the joints. It may affect any joint but is common in the smaller joints of the feet and hands. An acute attack may awaken a sufferer with pain in the big toe.

Non-Pain Related Medical Causes of Insomnia

Prostatic enlargement is a cause of insomnia in elderly males. Its symptoms are a frequency of urination at night, straining to urinate, and a reduced force of urination. It can occasionally lead to a sudden inability to urinate accompanied by severe bladder pain caused by distension. This necessitates immediate surgery. Frequent urination may also occur with infections of the urinary tract, inflammation of the kidney, bladder tumors, and in congestive heart failure.

The distress of **asthma** commonly occurs at night and frequently results in awakening with chest tightness, coughing, and wheezing. Attacks occur spontaneously or as a result of various trigger factors such as irritants (dusts, odors, smoke fumes), emotional stress, infection, physical exertion, changes in the weather, and allergies. The aminophyllines, and salbutamol used in the treatment of asthma are stimulants of the central nervous system and cause insomnia (chapter 21). We have shown that nocturnal asthma is triggered in part by REM sleep.

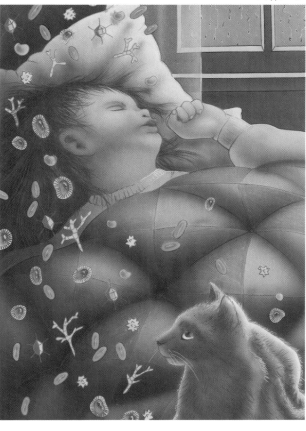

Figure 15-3
Many environmental factors influence nocturnal asthma, e.g., house-dust mites (Appendix)

Croup is an acute infection of the upper airways of the lung commonly arising at night with difficult breathing, a barking cough, and high fever. A seated position and cool air relieve the distress. A humidifier in the bedroom of the child is often helpful.

Allergies of the upper respiratory tract (e.g., hay fever) may cause severe nasal congestion, sneezing, and headaches disrupting sleep. House-dust mites (Figure 15-3), down filled bedding, and animal hair or dander are common causes of nighttime attacks. Use a foam mattress or a mattress

79

cover to prevent the growth of house-dust mites. Allergies affecting the skin, especially hives and eczema, produce intense itchiness which can seriously disrupt sleep.

Chronic lung disease with shortness of breath and cough may cause insomnia. In severe cases additional oxygen may be needed, especially at night, for the patient who may be confused, irritable, and severely distressed by a lack of sleep. These diseases include chronic bronchitis, emphysema, chronic obstructive airway disease, cystic fibrosis, and fibrosing alveolitis.

Nasal stuffiness from a variety of causes can be treated with, for example, Nasocort. Attention to the humidity in the home is important as dry air may lead to nasal stuffiness and nocturnal nose bleeds in children. Too much humidity leads to mite proliferation.

Nocturnal leg cramps commonly present with restless legs and cramps at night. This can be treated by clonazepam, clobazam, L-Dopa, selegiline hydrochloride, or codeine. These drugs require careful monitoring.

Patients with **Diabetes** on treatment sometimes awaken at night with tremors, headaches, sweating, slurring of speech, and blurred vision and may progress to coma. This occurs when an incorrect dose of medication, usually insulin, has been taken, or after an improper meal.

Kidney disease is associated with periodic leg movements during sleep which may cause sleep disruption.

This is only a general account of physically-related sleep problems, but it does cover the major medical (non-psychological) causes of sleep disruption.

Other Sleep Disorders That Cause Insomnia

here are several primary sleep disorders that can give rise to symptoms of insomnia. In sleep apnea, a person stops breathing for anywhere from a number of seconds to a couple of minutes, repeatedly, during the night. Sufferers are unaware of their problem so it is useful to question the bed partner about snoring or startling as this is sometimes related to sleep apnea. Occasional pauses in breathing during sleep are perfectly normal. When these pauses occur more than ten times per hour and last longer than ten seconds, this could be a sign of significant sleep apnea. As the pauses in breathing become longer, carbon dioxide levels in the blood are increasing (hypercapnia), while oxygen is decreasing (hypoxia). Subconscious responses are elicited to protect the brain from hypoxia. Apneas with arousals can produce symptoms of insomnia, without the individual knowing why he is awakening. These repetitive arousals may be so brief that the person does not remember any awakenings. He could think he slept soundly and wonder why he feels exhausted and sleepy throughout the day. Some of the characteristics of the "typical" patient with sleep apnea are shown in Figure 16-1.

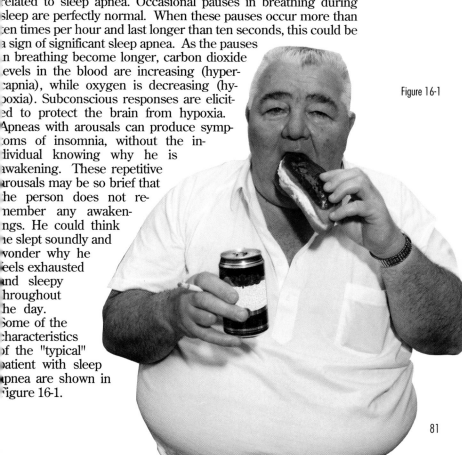

Figure 16-1

Table 16 lists commonly associated features of sleep apnea. Circle "yes" or "no". Not every person with sleep apnea has all of these. However, if you have any of the first three features and several of the others, you should ask your family doctor to refer you to a sleep specialist.

TABLE 16
CLINICAL FEATURES OF OBSTRUCTIVE SLEEP APNEA

Date: _____ Height : _____ Weight : _____

Neck Size: _____ Body Fat: _____ BMI: _____

Snoring	Yes	No
Excessive daytime sleepiness	Yes	No
Witnessed apneas	Yes	No
Other nocturnal features:		
Restless sleep	Yes	No
Choking	Yes	No
Enuresis (bed wetting)	Yes	No
Impotence (men only):		
Achieving Erection	Yes	No
Maintaining Erection	Yes	No
Esophageal reflux (heart burn)	Yes	No
Nightmares	Yes	No
Unrefreshing sleep	Yes	No
Other daytime features:		
Morning headache	Yes	No
Intellectual changes:		
Memory	Yes	No
Concentration	Yes	No
Personality changes	Yes	No
Lack of energy during the day	Yes	No
Morning confusion	Yes	No
Depression	Yes	No
Daytime naps	Yes	No
Associated conditions:		
Obesity	Yes	No
Hypertension (high blood pressure)	Yes	No
Large neck (17" or more in men)	Yes	No
Nasal obstruction	Yes	No
Jaw/nose surgery/fracture/abnormality	Yes	No
Hypothyroidism	Yes	No
Post-traumatic stress disorder	Yes	No
Post-menopausal (women only)	Yes	No
Recent weight gain	Yes	No
Do you have diabetes or chronic bronchitis?	Yes	No
Have you ever had a family member with sleep apnea?	Yes	No
Have you ever had a family member who died in his/her sleep?	Yes	No
Past history of muscular activity/competitive sports	Yes	No
Past history of heavy alcohol consumption	Yes	No

Snoring is a rattling of the soft tissues of the upper airway most often occurring as you breathe in. It is often associated with apnea, but you can certainly snore without having pauses in your breathing. Snoring can disturb the sleep of the snorer, but more often it plagues those within earshot.

Simple treatments include:

•Training yourself to sleep in a different position. If you snore more while sleeping on your back, put one or two tennis balls in an athletic sock and pin it to the back of your pyjamas. More elaborate devices, such as an anti-snoring pillow, are also available (Appendix).

•Drinking less alcohol. Snoring is less severe when no alcohol is consumed.

•Losing weight. Snoring usually increases with body weight.

•Providing ear plugs for the bed partner when all else fails.

Periodic leg movement during sleep (nocturnal myoclonus) is characterized by repetitive, periodic leg kicks during sleep. This should not be confused with "hypnic jerks" which startle some of us as we fall asleep. In this condition patients will twitch the muscles, particularly in their legs, with regular frequency throughout much of the night. A person may twitch his leg every 20 to 40 seconds for a period of one or two hours during the night, stop for a while, then resume twitching. The effect is to slightly but repeatedly disrupt sleep. It is like someone is shaking you on the shoulder gently so that you do not become fully awake. Often the person is totally unaware of this behavior. Sufferers usually find their bedclothes in disarray in the morning, with the sensation of a restless and disturbed sleep. Again, the bed partner is often just as disturbed from being on the receiving end of this relentless kicking.

Restless Legs Syndrome (RLS) is a waking phenomenon where there are sensations of restlessness in the legs, commonly associated with creeping and crawling sensations rather than with pain. The need to move or rub the legs constantly gives rise to severe insomnia. People with RLS tend to choose aisle seats on planes and in movie theaters.

Narcolepsy is characterized by irresistible daytime sleepiness, hallucinations on going to sleep or at awakening, and periods of full or partial paralysis on or after awakening. However, another important aspect of narcolepsy is the common complaint of insomnia. Improving the nocturnal sleep of narcoleptics can often lead to a reduction of medications required to alleviate daytime symptoms.

CHAPTER SEVENTEEN

Decison Trees to Help Identify the Causes of your Insomnia

When you have difficulty falling asleep there is often more than one cause. Tackling one aspect may not lead to a complete solution. It is necessary to correct each factor or you may continue to suffer sleep disturbance.

In this chapter there is a decision tree (Figure 17-1) designed to point to possible causes of your sleep disruption. The branches indicate various reasons for the type of sleep disruption you have. Possible solutions are indicated at the end of each branch. Recall that one particular problem can cause different types of sleep disruption. For example, someone who is depressed may have difficulty falling asleep, or may have early morning awakening. Thus some of the branches belong on more than one stem or main branch, which accounts for the linking between branches. You should consider yourself on each of the main stems, since you may have a problem falling asleep which is shown in Stem 1 (green), as well as a problem in the daytime which is shown in Stem 2 (orange). The solutions offered are not necessarily the only ones and other issues in your particular case may be important. For example, if you have difficulty falling asleep, one possible reason is anxiety, and one solution might be taking a sleeping medication. If you have had a drug or alcohol problem previously, such a solution may be much less desirable. The careful balancing of such information is best done by a clinician familiar with you, your problem, and the field of insomnia.

There are many aspects to the anxiety branch and it is possible that some twigs are missing. Anxiety may differ from one person to another. A second tree (Figure 17-2) shows some of the considerations in the case of anxiety. You should read the second decision tree to get a sense of the selections that may apply to your problem. A self-help book such as this has its limitations; however, you will identify more problems than might usually be the case. The average family doctor, when seeing a person with insomnia, asks only two or three questions before making a decision about treatment. In going through these decision trees you will ask more than 50 questions and will

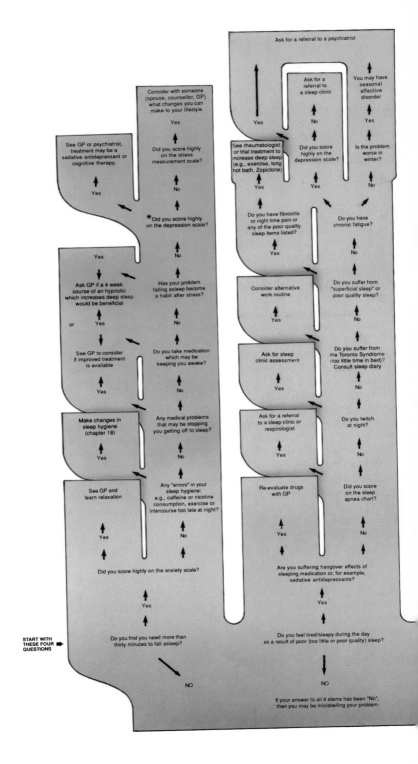

Ask for a referral to a psychiatrist

Ask for a referral to a sleep clinic ← Yes ← No → You may have seasonal affective disorder ← Yes

Consider with someone (spouse, counsellor, GP) what changes you can make to your lifestyle

Yes

See GP or psychiatrist, treatment may be a sedative antidepressant or cognitive therapy.

Yes

Did you score highly on the stress measurement scale?

No

See rheumatologist, or trial treatment to increase deep sleep (e.g., exercise, long hot bath, Zopiclone)

Did you score highly on the depression scale?

Yes

Is the problem worse in winter?

No

★Did you score highly on the depression scale?

No

Do you have fibrositis or night time pain or any of the poor quality sleep items listed?

Yes

Do you have chronic fatigue?

No

Yes

Ask GP if a 4 week course of an hypnotic which increases deep sleep would be beneficial

or   Yes

Has your problem falling asleep become a habit after stress?

No

Consider alternative work routine

Yes

Do you suffer from "superficial sleep" or poor quality sleep?

No

See GP to consider if improved treatment is available

Yes

Do you take medication which may be keeping you awake?

No

Ask for sleep clinic assessment

Yes

Do you suffer from the Toronto Syndrome (too little time in bed)? Consult sleep diary

No

Make changes in sleep hygiene (chapter 18)

Yes

Any medical problems that may be stopping you getting off to sleep?

No

Ask for a referral to a sleep clinic or respirologist

Yes

Do you twitch at night?

No

See GP and learn relaxation

Yes

Any "errors" in your sleep hygiene: e.g., caffeine or nicotine consumption, exercise or intercourse too late at night?

No

Re-evaluate drugs with GP

Yes

Did you score on the sleep apnea chart?

No

Did you score highly on the anxiety scale?

Yes

Are you suffering hangover effects of sleeping medication or, for example, sedative antidepressants?

Yes

START WITH THESE FOUR QUESTIONS ➡ Do you find you need more than thirty minutes to fall asleep?

NO

Do you feel tired/sleepy during the day as a result of poor (too little or poor quality) sleep?

NO

If your answer to all 4 stems has been "No", then you may be mislabelling your problem

86

Figure 17-1
A decision tree
to help you explore
various causes and
possible treatments
of your insomnia

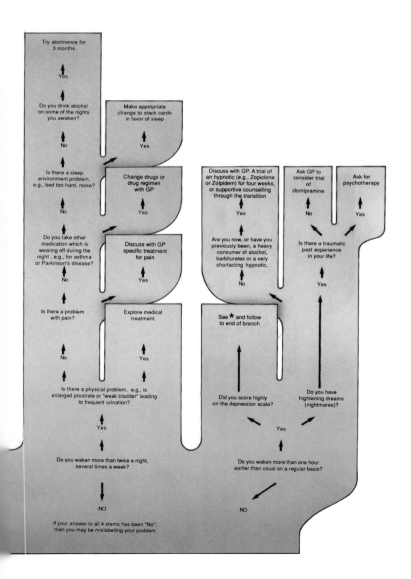

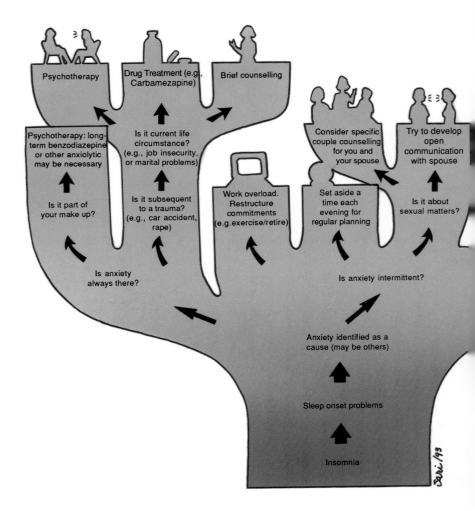

Psychotherapy

Drug Treatment (e.g., Carbamezapine)

Brief counselling

Psychotherapy: long-term benzodiazepine or other anxiolytic may be necessary

Is it current life circumstance? (e.g., job insecurity, or marital problems)

Consider specific couple counselling for you and your spouse

Try to develop open communication with spouse

Is it part of your make up?

Is it subsequent to a trauma? (e.g., car accident, rape)

Work overload. Restructure commitments (e.g.exercise/retire)

Set aside a time each evening for regular planning

Is it about sexual matters?

Is anxiety always there?

Is anxiety intermittent?

Anxiety identified as a cause (may be others)

Sleep onset problems

Insomnia

Sari/93

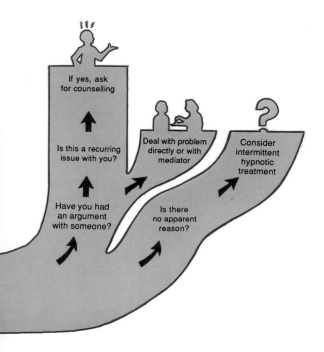

If yes, ask
for counselling

Is this a recurring
issue with you?

Deal with problem
directly or with
mediator

Consider
intermittent
hypnotic
treatment

Have you had
an argument
with someone?

Is there
no apparent
reason?

Figure 17-2
A decision tree
showing some causes
and possible treatments
of anxiety-related insomnia

89

therefore achieve a more sophisticated understanding of your problem. Completion of the other questionnaires and the sleep diary will add enormously to your knowledge about your insomnia.

If you get on with your assessment without "playing doctor" you can then have a more informed discussion with your family physician about treatment options, or at least encourage your doctor to refer you to a specialist, if appropriate.

For any particular problem there may be a range of different solutions: changes in sleep hygiene; behavioral changes; counselling; medication, either for sleeping or for treatment of other conditions; medical treatment; or obtaining more information. Some of these are discussed in the following chapter.

One option that is often overlooked is the use of self-help organizations. If you think you have seasonal affective disorder, chronic fatigue, or a sleep-related problem, there are specific self-help groups to consider. Addresses are given in the Appendix. Joining such organizations allows you to keep in touch with new developments regarding your problem. In many cases, sleep problems are only *mostly* solved, rather than *completely* solved, and may recur. A self-help group allows you to realize that your problems are not unique. There is comfort in learning how others cope.

CHAPTER EIGHTEEN

Sleep Hygiene Rules

Sleep Schedule

Adhering to a consistent schedule of sleeping and waking is one of the most important rules of proper sleep hygiene. This is especially important for individuals who are sensitive or susceptible to disruptions in their sleep-wake cycle. Elimination of daytime naps, consistent scheduling of meals, elimination of caffeine and alcohol in the evening, consistent bedtime, and adequate allowance for sleep time can become the cycle of health. Though difficult, you can move the hands of your biological clock to suit the schedule of your own environment. This will ensure adequate and efficient sleep resulting in daytime alertness and a feeling of well-being.

Shift workers have specific problems. Inappropriate sleep-wake schedules are imposed on the shift worker by the demands of this working environment. Beginning a night shift, he arrives home in the morning and goes to bed when the rest of the world is coming to life. He attempts to sleep when all body functions are expecting a waking episode. His sleep is fragmented, disturbed, and unrefreshing. Even if he arrives home and sleeps a normal length of time, his sleep usually lacks restorative quality. Some people adapt to shift work with no problems, but it becomes increasingly difficult as they age. These tips can make their lives much easier.

- As it takes several days to adapt to a new shift, longer shifts are preferable to shorter ones.
- Shift rotation should be clockwise: you should move from day, to afternoon, to night shifts, rather than the reverse. The biological clock prefers to shift to a later time rather than to an earlier one.
- Shift workers should have regular meal times with breakfast, lunch, and dinner corresponding to the shift schedule. The quality and quantity of food should correspond to that eaten while not working shifts.
- Nighttime workers who have 90 minutes of sleep mid-shift adapt much better to night work and maintain synchronized biological rhythms.

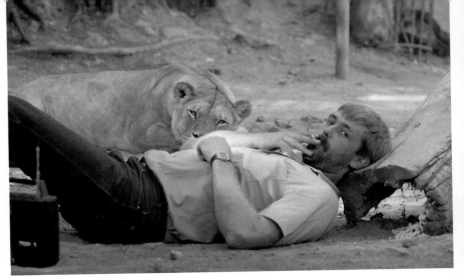

Figure 18-1
Certain circumstances (as well as smoking) are not conducive to sleep

Sleep Environment (Figure 18-1)

Aspects of your physical surroundings have a strong influence on how well you sleep. Examine your environment carefully to decide what factors are important to *your* sleep.

Noise means different things to different people. Some may sleep through thunderstorms but awaken easily to a child's cry. Some enjoy complete quiet, while others prefer a constant noise such as an air conditioner. Loud, sudden noise disturbs sleep even in people who do not awaken. If loud noise is a problem for you it may be worthwhile to consider soundproofing, noise screening, or earplugs.

No specific **temperature** has been found to be ideal. Too cold (below 17°C or 65°F) or too hot (above 24°C or 80°F) seem

Figure 18-2
A long, hot bath before sleep and a cool sleeping environment may facilitate sleep onset

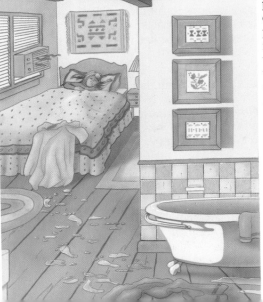

to inhibit sleep. Cold temperatures cause unpleasant dreams whereas hot temperatures may cause people to move more in their sleep and to wake up more often. Explore what temperature allows you to sleep best. Adjusting your night attire may make a difference. Using a fan may provide a noise screen as well as a temperature modulator. Plugging the fan into a timer will allow a cooler period earlier in the night, should this be desirable. The last thing you want to do is to wake up three hours into your sleep to switch off a fan. When you dream during REM sleep, you cannot control your body temperature.

Sweating stops even in a hot environment and shivering stops even if it is cold.

During the first deep sleep episode body temperature steadily falls. Raising body temperature with a long hot bath or sauna, and ensuring a cool environment at sleep onset, allow the body temperature to fall facilitating sleep (Figure 18-2). Daytime heating facilitates sleep; but, if the bedding environment is heated after sleep begins, sleep is disrupted.

You may find you sleep better with or without a **bed partner** (Figure 18-3), or with or without a dog. Some are disturbed by the movement or noise, whereas others enjoy the emotional comfort. Some find twin beds preferable to a double bed. If your sleep problem is leading to your sleeping in different a bedroom, referral to a sleep clinic is indicated.

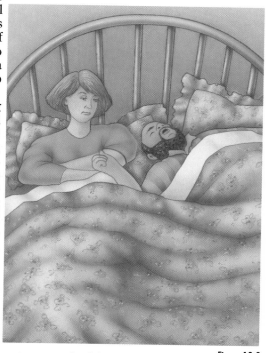

Figure 18-3
Tensions in a relationship can disrupt sleep

The only truism regarding **beds** is that an excessively hard surface (e.g., wooden floor) disturbs sleep. People have an enormous range of bed preferences. It is important for you to explore what surface is best for you. Back pain at night is not always helped by a hard bed! However, better quality mattresses are usually associated with long-term comfort.

Examine your sleep **environment** for disturbances that are beyond your control. The continual disruption of sleep by small children can often result in "learned" insomnia. Unlearning bad habits may require specific treatment and advice from your doctor.

Substances:
The Do's and Don'ts of Food, Drink, and Medication

• Losing or gaining weight has a surprisingly great influence on sleep. Weight gain results in longer, undisturbed sleep whereas weight loss or dieting may cause sleep disruption. For those with sleep apnea weight loss will usually improve sleep.
• Over-the-counter sleep aids often contain antihistamines. They should generally be avoided. While they can cause drowsiness,

93

some people may become over-stimulated. If you use a drug to promote sleep onset, use a prescription drug made specifically for the purpose.

• In general, sleeping pills should not be taken for more than four weeks. Regular use can actually increase insomnia. If you have been taking sleeping pills for some time it is important to plan the process of withdrawal. Some doctors recommend decreasing intake gradually to compensate for the physiological dependence. This applies only if a person has been on high doses or on tranquilizers and sleeping pills concurrently. Abrupt switching from benzodiazepines to Zopiclone for four weeks and then stopping all drugs is a successful method we have used to help patients stop taking sleeping pills (Figure 14-1). Some insomniacs require drug treatment, usually for a period of three to four weeks. However, there are important exceptions. Consult your doctor.

• Reduce most fluids after dinner time, to avoid the need to urinate in the middle of the night. Try a glass of milk at night. It is a natural source of tryptophan, an amino acid helpful in inducing sleep. Other useful drinks are Ovaltine and Horlicks. A major factor determining the impact of a pre-bed snack is how regularly you eat or drink before bedtime. A habit or ritual is an important aid to sleep onset.

• Avoid caffeine in the late afternoon and evening. Caffeine is a natural stimulant with a dramatic effect on sleep. Avoid coffee, tea, colas, and chocolate (Table 14).

• Avoid late evening alcohol consumption. It may help you to fall asleep but it actually disturbs sleep patterns and can cause early morning or even middle of the night awakening, especially if you are more than 40 years old. Sleep disruption (even undetected) at an earlier age may have an impact on sleep later in life.

• Smoking reduces sleep duration by 30 minutes per night on average (Figure 18-1).

• Certain other drugs may interfere with sleep (e.g., drugs used for asthma and hypertension). If you are taking any other drugs regularly, ask your doctor about their possible effects on sleep.

Other Strategies
• Develop regular bedtime habits. Most insomniacs stay in bed too long and/or get up too late in the morning after a poor night. Get up at the same time each day even if you're tired.

• If you wake up at night, try to remain in bed and relax. If you feel yourself becoming tense and frustrated don't just lie there. Read, if this relaxes you, or get up and enjoy a quiet activity to prepare yourself for sleep again after about 20 minutes. Give yourself about 30 minutes in bed before repeating this cycle.

• Use an alarm clock to wake you at your regular time, but position it away from you so you don't "clock watch" which can cause unnecessary tension.

• If naps upset your regular night's sleep don't take them. There are exceptions where daytime napping may help sleep the next night.

• If daily naps are a good thing for you then have one every day or not at all. People who occasionally nap often find that they usually do not sleep well the same night.

• Exercise is very important if you want to develop good sleep habits. Exercise regularly in the morning or in the early afternoon. Avoid strenuous physical activity in the late evening; this time should always be associated with quiet activity. Keep yourself fit even if you're tired from insomnia. Healthy bodies sleep better than unfit ones. If you currently do no exercise, start gently. For example, begin by swimming three or four pool lengths the first day and increase the rate by two lengths every second day. Within a month you will notice a clear effect on your sleep. Most successful approaches to sleep problems are gradual as this example illustrates. Do not expect an abrupt change.

• Save your bedroom for sex and sleep. Learn to associate your bedroom with sleep-related activities only. This will help you to sleep when you get into bed at night. Don't study, watch TV, or eat in bed unless these *directly* help you to fall asleep. At the same time, avoid sleeping in other places around your house or apartment.

• Develop daily bedtime habits. These will remind you that it is time for sleep. For example, you may start by locking your doors and closing your windows. Then take a warm bath or shower, brush your teeth, change into your sleep wear, turn down your bed, set your alarm clock, practice a relaxation technique or meditate, and turn off the lights. Do whatever works for you, but do the same thing every night.

• Learn to associate lying in bed with a relaxed mind. If you go to bed and find yourself worrying about things, get out of bed and do a quiet activity. It is better to go to bed when you're drowsy.

• If worrying keeps you awake, set aside a fifteen minute "worry" period to occur at the same time, perhaps after dinner, and in the same place every day. Be strict and make sure you do all your worrying in this time and think *intently* about your concerns. Remind yourself about this "worry period" if you wake up trying to solve your problems in the middle of the night. Remember, too, that you're not really alert enough to resolve problems when you're half asleep.

• Learn to relax your body. If you are tense, deep-muscle relaxation will help. Clench your fists, feel the tension for a few short seconds, then quickly relax your abdominal area, and finally your legs. Take deep, slow, rhythmic breaths to help you relax. There are audio tapes designed to aid relaxation (Appendix).

• Don't label yourself an "insomniac". Most people have difficulty sleeping now and then. This is normal. If you call yourself an insomniac, you could develop problems simply because you expect to.

• Worrying about insomnia is often more of a problem than the insomnia itself. Take note of your thoughts during a bad night and try to substitute positive thoughts about your sleep for negative ones. Consistent substitution often results in their occurring naturally. A person who tells himself "I must get a good night's sleep otherwise I will be a wreck tomorrow" is more likely to suffer insomnia than one who thinks, "If I don't sleep tonight I will still be able to function".

• Certain physical symptoms may interfere with your sleep (e.g., a cough, toothache). If you experience physical symptoms that disturb your sleep consult your doctor.

• Don't allow yourself too much time in bed. Especially among the elderly, restricting time in bed to the hours of sleep, and then adding 15-30 minutes per week, is a helpful strategy for increasing sleep time.

There are many recommendations listed in this chapter. Focus on two or three that seem most applicable to you. After a few weeks, reread this chapter to evaluate your success in making the changes you chose and to see if there are any others to be made.

CHAPTER NINETEEN

Tips for Getting Off to Sleep

We have previously outlined some general rules on nighttime procedure for people with insomnia. Here are some specific, practical ideas to help you drift off to sleep. Some have been mentioned before.

General Pointers

• Don't punish yourself with thinking which leads nowhere. For example, "I should be sleeping", "I'll never function tomorrow if I don't fall asleep now!" Shakespeare's approach in *As You Like It*, "I'll go to sleep if I can; if I cannot, I'll rail against all the first-born of Egypt", was wrong.

• Occupy your thoughts and body with predetermined tasks for getting off to sleep, e.g., counting sheep and relaxation exercises.

• Choose pre-sleep activities that you can leave at any time. For example, don't read a book that you simply have to finish.

• Set yourself the unusual goal of discovering which activities are the most uninteresting to you. Do these before going to bed so that sleep seems an attractive alternative.

Specific Pointers

Here are some ideas for a boring night. All are done while lying in bed. You may find some of your own to add to this list. Choose one suggestion only!

• "Counting sheep" is the oldest trick in the book but it still has merit. Counting or visualizing anything repetitively will have a similar effect. Repetition, by its very nature, is unstimulating and hypnotic.

- Go around your home (in your mind's eye) straightening all the pictures and when you've finished, start again.

- Story rituals. Create an ending to a movie or compose a short story on the same theme. Repeat the same story every night.

- Visualize yourself in a tranquil scene, feeling totally relaxed, with nothing on your mind but taking in what you see, perhaps a mountain scene or calm lake.

- Squint your eyes in the dim light and focus on an object in the room. Try to close your eyes as much as possible while keeping focused on the object you can barely see. Empty your mind of all else but the object. For some people who feel tired, closing their eyes switches on all sorts of thoughts of things they should do. This technique will help eliminate this problem.

- Read a boring book, which you have put aside previously for this purpose. It must be a book which can be put down at any stage.

- Design your dream house in your mind.

- Think of five things you can see in your room, five things you can hear, and five things you are aware of. Repeat the above with four items in each category. If you cannot think of new items, you can reuse the old ones. Repeat with three, two, and then one item in each category. This exercise is boring enough that you will drift off to sleep but sufficiently complex to keep you engaged without allowing your mind to wander off onto other exciting or anxiety-provoking thoughts.

- Visualize a blackboard. Anything that comes on — rub it off!

If you are unable to sleep after 30 minutes of trying one of the previous suggestions get out of bed and try one of these activities:

- Make a list of all your concerns then put them aside to deal with the following day. This is usually better done in the early evening.

- Watch a boring movie. The same "book" rules apply here.

- Organize and rewrite your recipe box or address book. One tends to postpone these tasks, so this will be time well spent albeit a boring time.

- Organize your photo albums. Take all your packets of photos and put them in chronological order.

- Listen to soothing music or a relaxation tape.

- Take a warm bath if this relaxes you.

- Do any repetitive task such as knitting, needlepoint, dusting your book shelf, or straightening your closets.

Hopefully, some of these suggestions will help you fall back to sleep. Even if they don't achieve this immediately, you will at least have spent your time awake positively and productively.

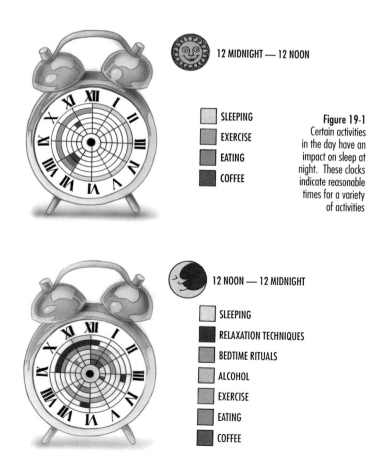

12 MIDNIGHT — 12 NOON

☐ SLEEPING
☐ EXERCISE
☐ EATING
■ COFFEE

Figure 19-1
Certain activities in the day have an impact on sleep at night. These clocks indicate reasonable times for a variety of activities

12 NOON — 12 MIDNIGHT

☐ SLEEPING
■ RELAXATION TECHNIQUES
☐ BEDTIME RITUALS
☐ ALCOHOL
☐ EXERCISE
☐ EATING
■ COFFEE

CHAPTER TWENTY

Behavioral Strategies for Improved Sleep

Numerous behavioral techniques have been shown effective in the management of insomnia. The choice of the technique will depend on the nature of the problem. If you are able to "self-assess" your sleep problem with the help of this book, it should not be difficult for you to select treatment strategies to suit your particular needs. Each section in this chapter will identify the *PROBLEM* (certain sleep problems), which will be followed by the *SOLUTION* (behavioral interventions).

PROBLEM: *Inadequate sleep hygiene* is a sleep disorder resulting from daytime activities which affect quality of sleep and subsequent daytime performance. These include: irregular sleep-wake schedule, restricting time allocated for sleep, exercise close to bedtime, intense mental work late at night, partying late at night, clock-watching during the night, inappropriate ambient temperature, pets in the bedroom, excessive daytime napping, use of hypnotics/alcohol to promote sleep, and excessive caffeine intake.

SOLUTION: *Sleep Hygiene Rules* Discussed in chapter 18, these are the bases for improving sleep. Here we place these rules in the context of overcoming specific problems.
- Do not go to bed until you are drowsy.
- Get up at approximately the same time each morning even on weekends. If you want to sleep in on the weekend, allow yourself only one extra hour in bed.
- Do not take naps.

These three rules will give you a consistent sleep rhythm and synchronize your biologic clock. In time, your bedtime, or the time when you become drowsy, will also tend to become regular.
- Do not drink alcohol less than two hours before bedtime.

- Do not consume caffeine after about 4:00 p.m., or in the six hours prior to bedtime. Become familiar with the foods, beverages, and medications that contain caffeine (chapter 14).
- Do not smoke within several hours of your bedtime.
- Exercise regularly. The best time to exercise is early in the day. Avoid strenuous physical exertion after 6:00 p.m.
- Use common sense to make your sleep environment most conducive to sleep. Arrange for a comfortable temperature and minimum levels of sound, light, and noise.
- If you are accustomed to it, have a light carbohydrate or dairy snack before bedtime (e.g., crackers, graham crackers, milk, cheese). Do not eat chocolate or large amounts of sugar. Avoid excessive fluids. If you awaken in the middle of the night, do not have a snack or you may find that you begin to wake up habitually at that time feeling hungry.

PROBLEM: *Insomnia in the presence of adequate sleep hygiene.* If you follow the rules of good sleep hygiene but still have difficulty sleeping other factors must be considered. Your wake drive may be too strong or your sleep drive too weak. You may have been born with this inadequacy. If this is the case some extra work may be required.

SOLUTION: *Stimulus control* Some of the following instructions overlap with others already presented. However, the specific goal of these "stimulus control" instructions is to help you develop sleep habits that will facilitate falling asleep and staying asleep by strengthening any stimulus which promotes sleep while weakening any stimulus incompatible with sleep.
- Lie down and try to sleep only when you are sleepy.
- Do not use your bed for anything except sleep or sex; do not read, watch television, do homework, pay bills, eat, or worry in bed.
- If you find yourself unable to sleep, get up and go into another room. Stay up as long as you wish and then return to the bedroom to sleep when you become drowsy. Although you should not watch the clock, get out of bed again if you do not fall asleep within approximately 30 minutes. If you do not fall asleep, repeat this step as often as necessary throughout the night.
- Set your alarm and get up at the same time every morning, irrespective of how much sleep you had the previous night. This will help your body acquire a consistent sleep rhythm. Knowing

that your alarm is set, and that you will not miss that important "wake up" signal, turn your clock around so that you cannot read the time. Do not look at the clock until the alarm goes off. This will be difficult, but avoid temptation. Clock watching can be a major source of stress during the night.

• Do not nap during the day.

SOLUTION: *Sleep restriction* can be tried on its own or in conjunction with any other suggested strategies. After completing the sleep diary (chapter 6), you can estimate your average sleep length, as well as the time you most often fall asleep and awaken. Use this information to create a schedule.

For example, if you estimate that you take three hours to get to sleep and only get four hours of sleep before your alarm goes off, then this becomes your new schedule. If you go to bed at 11:00 p.m., but don't fall asleep until 2:00 a.m., you now start going to bed at 2:00 a.m., but still get up at your usual time. You have taken control by saying to your brain, "If all you're going to give me is four hours of sleep, then that's all I'm going to allow". If after a period of one week you are sleeping (on most nights) for 90 percent of the time you are in bed, but still feeling poorly during the day, then it is time to expand the sleep period to allow for an expanding sleep time. The general rule is to allow 15 to 30 minutes extra per week. You just may find that your sleep expands to fill the time allowed, eventually providing sleep that is adequate in both length and efficiency.

PROBLEM: *Worry, stress, anxiety.* These can all interfere with your ability to sleep by keeping you in a constant state of alertness. The object is to reduce alertness and arousability by attempting to establish a hypometabolic, deeply relaxed state. By achieving a state of deep relaxation upon going to bed, you are more likely to fall asleep quickly and stay asleep.

SOLUTION: *Progressive muscle relaxation (PMR).* Psychological stress often manifests itself as a series of unpleasant physical sensations, such as heart palpitations, excessive sweating, butterflies in the stomach, headache, and a stiff neck. Often the stress escalates as the brain identifies these bodily reactions giving way to a vicious cycle. By reducing blood pressure, heart rate, breathing rate, muscular tensions, and perspiration, you can effectively limit the impact of environmental stress.

Mastering relaxation techniques can be like having a built-in anti-anxiety pill. Most people do not appreciate muscular tension, and certainly have no idea which of their muscles is chronically tense. PMR isolates particular muscle groups and allows you to distinguish between sensations of tension and relaxation within those muscles.

The major muscle groups are: hands, forearms, and biceps; head and face (forehead, eyes, nose, cheeks, lips, jaws) and the neck and shoulders (considerable attention is devoted to the head, neck, and shoulders as these areas are very reactive to emotional tides); chest, stomach, and lower back; thigh, buttocks, calves, and feet.

Practice PMR either lying down or sitting in a chair. Each muscle group should be tensed for five to ten seconds, then relaxed for 20 to 30 seconds. Feel the tension and discomfort in the contracted muscle, and let the tension go by allowing the muscle group to completely relax. Feel the warmth and comfort that comes with relaxation. A little practice every day can make this technique more "portable", that is, it can be done quickly anywhere, anytime. Next time you are in a traffic jam, focus on the muscles of your neck. You will probably notice that your shoulders are raised and your neck stiff. Let go of the tension (while driving) and appreciate the difference. Adjusting your level of tension throughout the day can significantly influence your pattern of sleep.

For many, the best way to practice is by listening to a tape recording by a sleep therapist prior to bed time. These tapes are commercially available (Appendix), and will guide you through the most important muscle groups.

SOLUTION: In *Guided imagery* you use your imagination to provide relaxation. This is especially effective as you try to fall asleep.

Identify an image or activity most pleasing to you. Imagine a location, object, person, memory or fantasy that is pleasing to you such as a forest, a beach, snow falling, a hobby, or an accomplishment that was rewarding. One woman imagined winning a lottery, and then focused on all the wonderful things she could do for those around her with her windfall.

Whatever your image, settle into your scene by imagining sounds, smells, textures, colors and sensations. If you aim to maintain your image for at least 20 minutes without allowing the intrusion of stressful or stimulating thoughts, you will probably be asleep before 20 minutes are up. Commercial tape recordings are effective as demonstrations of the technique.

SOLUTION: *Biofeedback* is intended to help make you aware of body processes of which you were previously unconscious.

Specialized electronic equipment gives you immediate information about your biological state such as muscle tension, heart rate, sweating rate, surface skin temperature, and even brain wave activity.

If muscle tension is presented as a constant tone, with the tone becoming louder or softer as muscle tension increases and decreases, by trial and error, you can learn which "buttons" in your brain control the tension. The same applies to your heart rate. You can actually learn how to slow your own heart. After practice you can control these body functions without the aid of the machine.

This is obviously a more cumbersome, expensive, and labor-intensive technique than the others, and should be used advisedly.

PROBLEM: *Conquering the "All I may try, I will not succeed" attitude.* This may be based on previous half-hearted attempts at dealing with the problem, or on dealing only with part of the problem at any one time.

It may be that you are so concerned about your poor sleep that this concern has taken on wider dimensions and you feel generally depressed. Many types of unresolved or relentless stress can lead to depression. Insomnia is an important cause as well as consequence of depression.

SOLUTION: *Cognitive behavioral treatment.* This is a new technique used by psychologists for treating depression. It has also been found to be effective in the management of insomnia.

This is not a "do it yourself" technique. If you feel this approach may suit you, you should ask your family doctor to refer you to a specialized sleep clinic or a psychologist who uses this technique.

Its basic premise is to challenge the assumptions that a person may have about his sleep. There may be exaggeration of the problem, "catastrophizing" the consequences, and mistaken beliefs about sleep itself. Typically, all of these would be discussed over a period of eight to ten therapy sessions.

These are only a few of many techniques aimed at reducing existing stress, promoting relaxation and sleep, and reducing your reaction to future stress. Table 20 lists the range of techniques used.

A great deal of material has been presented here on the behavioral management of insomnia. You must decide which of the principles discussed best apply to you. Perhaps elements from each category apply and can be selected accordingly. It is important to be open-minded. The response will not be immediate. You have to stick to new rules and practice new techniques for several weeks before you will be able to determine whether or not they are truly effective. Patience and discipline are essential.

Table 20: Behavioral Treatments for Insomnia

Autogenic Training
Systematically focus on specific muscle groups (e.g., arms, legs)to induce feelings of warmth or heaviness in those muscles.

Biofeedback
EMG: to relax specific muscles (usually frontalis).

Cognitive Therapy
to change false concepts and thinking patterns about sleep.

Desensitization
to sleep-disturbing and anxiety-arousing images. Associated with relaxation.

Hypnotic Relaxation
Person is given suggestion to relax. Hypnosis is not generally very effective.

Meditation
Focus on single mental stimulus (e.g., word, phrase, image, or sound) subvocalized repeatedly. Usually done prior to bedtime.

Metronome-Conditioned Relaxation
Subject listens to metronome each night upon retiring. Verbal relaxation instructions paired with sounds of metronome.

Progressive Muscle Relaxation (PMR)
Tense and relax specific muscle groups (e.g., forearms, biceps, neck) systematically; focus on feelings of relaxation. Usually done prior to bedtime.

Sleep Restriction

Initially cutting down the amount of time allowed for sleep and then gradually expanding sleep time.

Stimulus Control

Associate bed and bedroom only with sleep. In bedroom, eliminate or reduce activities incompatible with sleep while in bed and at bedtime. Person must leave bed and bedroom if not sleeping or engaged in sexual activity.

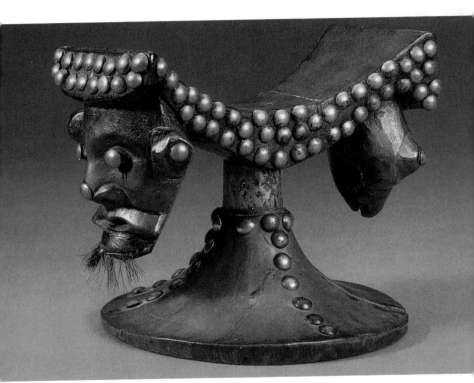

Figure 20-1
Many cultures have sleep aids.
This headrest may not appear comfortable to you, but it was actually used.
A regular routine and comfort are important components of behavioral treatment

CHAPTER TWENTY-ONE

Pharmacology of Hypnotics

Drugs Used in Insomnia
Drugs which promote sleep are called hypnotics. Some hypnotics have other effects and may also alleviate anxiety or foster muscle relaxation. They are used to promote sleep and to maintain daytime alertness.

The most popular hypnotic drugs prescribed in the 1950s for insomnia were the barbiturates. Tolerance and dependence increased consumption of the drug two-fold in one decade. In the 1960s, benzodiazepines (a safer group of drugs) were introduced. These are still popular. The 1990s have uncovered newer, more specific drugs of which Zopiclone (Imovane) and Zolpidem are examples.

There are many different groups of drugs used for promoting sleep (Table 21-1). Most are not purely hypnotic and should not be used as sleeping medications unless there is a very specific reason for doing so. We have indicated with an "X" those that should not be used only for the purpose of promoting sleep.

Table 21-1: Drugs that Promote Sleep

Sedative: Hypnotic
Barbiturates (Secobarbital) X
Glycerol derivative (Meprobamate - Equanol) X
Benzodiazepines (Ativan, Robinol, Valium)
Others: chloral hydrate, ethclorvynol, alcohol X
Cyclopyrrolone: Zopiclone (Imovane)
Imidazopyridine: Zolpidem

Sedative: Autonomic
Antihistamines (Benadryl, Atarax) X
Phenothiazine antipsychotics (Mellaril, chlorpromazine) X
Sedative tricyclic antidepressants (Doxepin, Sinequan) X
Azaspirodecandeione (Buspar) X

Sedative: Natural Substances
Tryptophan
Melatonin

All drugs which cause sedation act on nerve cells in the brain. Some act at very specific sites on specific cells but other compounds act more generally. The end result of this action is reduced anxiety, increased sleepiness, and relaxation of the muscles. Some drugs have a greater effect on reducing anxiety. Others have a greater effect on sleep.

The table on pages 110 and 111 lists the commonly used hypnotics. Most important from your perspective is the balance between the advantages and disadvantages of any drugs. These are carefully noted.

Many factors are taken into consideration in providing an appropriate hypnotic for a particular patient. In general, very long acting drugs may lead to sedation the next day.

Daytime sedation is less prominent in the very rapid-acting and intermediate-acting drugs. There is less accumulation of the drug in the body with this group. Zopiclone, Zolpidem, and Triazolam are excreted most quickly from the body. Flurazepam is long acting and has an active metabolite which is still in the body after 50 to 100 hours. In the elderly that may extend up to 300 hours. For this reason, the elderly should receive reduced dosages of certain hypnotic drugs — half or less of the usual adult dose. Very short acting drugs may cause rebound anxiety in the middle of the night. This is particulary so with Triazolam (Halcion). In general those drugs which act for the duration of the normal sleep period present fewest problems.

Pharmacology

After a drug is ingested it must be absorbed from the gut, distributed to the brain, inactivated, and then eliminated from the body.

The quicker it is absorbed the faster it exerts its effect. Sleep-inducing medications should be quickly absorbed. If not, the drug may have an effect long beyond the usual sleep period producing sleepiness the next day. Yet the drug has to remain long enough above a certain level in the body's tissues to maintain its effect. This level may differ with a person's age, weight, and body surface area. Older and thinner individuals require smaller doses hence the need for dose variation.

After absorption many drugs rapidly cross the blood/brain barrier and reach a steady level in the brain. Drugs with longer half-lives take longer to reach this steady level and to be eliminated from the body. Hence, they accumulate in the brain tissue. Drugs with a short half-life do not accumulate as much and are less likely to produce hangover effects in the morning. This is especially important in the elderly and in the ill individual. For some drugs, such as those used to treat anxiety or depression, an effective level may be reached only after a few days of taking the drug as it accumulates in the body. To determine an optimum dosage the drug must be taken regularly for a few days. Elimination of a drug by the body occurs by biotransformation (inactivation) and excretion through urine and bile. The half-life of a drug is the time it takes for half of the drug to be eliminated.

Some short acting drugs produce a rebound effect. This occurs soon after stopping the drug, producing a worse form of insomnia and anxiety. With the longer acting drug, this effect may be delayed for several days or may not occur because of a slow decline in blood levels.

Contraindications to Using Hypnotics

Hypnotics should not be used in the following circumstances.

•Pregnancy: Use may harm the fetus's organ formation and impair the baby's breathing at birth. Breast feeding is an even stronger contraindication.

•Unexplained daytime drowsiness: Avoid all sedatives and alcohol until a diagnosis has been made.

•Uncontrollable drug or alcohol abuse: There is a risk of hypnotic abuse. The combined effect of other drugs added to hypnotics may be life-threatening.

•A history of past hypnotic abuse.

•A history of unusual reaction to hypnotics not anticipated by the prescribing doctor.

Classes and Hypnotic Medications

Barbiturates: This class includes drugs such as Seconal, Nembutal, Secobarbital, Periobarbital, Amobarbital. These drugs are rarely used in insomnia today because of high risks of tolerance, dependence, addiction, and death by overdose. Alcohol greatly increases risk of the latter especially in alcoholic liver disease. Although very sedating, these drugs may actually worsen sleep and produce marked rebound insomnia associated with hallucinations, anxiety, and convulsions.

Other "Older" Drugs: These include meprobamate (Equanil), chloral hydrate (Noctec) and Ethclorvynol (Placidyl). They are all associated with rapid tolerance, physical dependence, and abuse and are dangerous in overdose. As with barbiturates, marked rebound insomnia upon discontinuation is typical.

Benzodiazepines: These drugs were introduced as sedatives in the 1960s. Flurazepam was the first benzodiazepine to be specifically indicated for sleep in 1974. In 1986 Triazolam (Halcion) became the most popular hypnotic.

Several problems were seen with their extensive use. These included tolerance to the drugs, withdrawal effects, physical and psychological dependence, and abuse. Most recently, amnesia

Table 21-2:

HYPNOTIC	USUAL DAILY DOSE	TIME (hrs) TO PEAK PLASMA LEVELS	DURATIO OF ACTIO
Diazepam (Valium, Vual, Meral)	5 - 10 mg	1	Long
Flurazepam (Dalmane, Paxane)	15 to 30 mg	0.5 to 1.5	Long
Lorazepam (Ativan)	1 - 2 mg	5 (oral), 0.25 (sub-lingual) 'under tongue'	Medium
Lormetazepam (Noctamide)	1 - 2 mg	1 - 2 (soft)	Medium
Nitrazepam (Mogadon)	2.25 to 5 mg	1 to 5	Long
Oxazepam (Serax, Zapex, Oxpam)	15 to 30 mg	2.2	Medium
Temazepam (Restoril, Normisan)	15 to 30 mg	2 to 3	Medium
Triazolam (Halcion)	0.125 to 0.25 mg	1 to 5	Very short
Zolpidem (Stillnox, Ambien)	10 mg	1	Very short
Zopiclone (Imovane, Amoban, Limovan, Xinovan, Zimovane)	3.75 to 7.5 mg	0.5 to 1.5	Short

Hypnotics — their assets and drawbacks

ASSETS	DRAWBACKS
• No withdrawal effects • Good for anxiety	• Slow elimination • Can accumulate with repeated dosing • Residual daytime effects
• Rapid onset of action • Suitable for initial, middle and late insomnia • Delayed tolerance • Minimal rebound insomnia • Daytime anxiolytic effect	• Accumulates with repeated dosing • Moderate "hangover" effects • Daytime sedation • Additive effects with alcohol and CNS depressants • Psychomotor impairments (e.g., increased reaction time) • Not suitable for the elderly
• Sub-lingual formulation • Very rapid absorption	• Slow and variable absorption • Clinical indication uncertain
2 formulations available	• May alter sleep architecture
• Rapid onset • Suitable for initial, middle, and late insomnia • Delayed tolerance • Minimal rebound insomnia • Daytime anxiolytic insomnia	• Accumulates with repeated dosing • Moderate "hangover" effects • Daytime sedation • Additive effects with alcohol and CNS depressants • Psychomotor impairments • Not suitable for the elderly
• Few hangover effects • Good for anxiety-related insomnia	• Slow onset of action
• Useful for middle and late insomnia • Does not accumulate • Few "hangover" effects • Minimal rebound insomnia • Minimal psychomotor impairment	• Slow onset of action • Additive effects with alcohol and CNS depressants
• Rapid onset • Does not accumulate Few "hangover" effects • No daytime sedation • Absence of psychomotor impairment	• Recent "bad press" which has lead to low patient acceptance • Tolerance within three weeks of continued use • Marked rebound insomnia after sudden withdrawal (related to duration of use and dose) • Can cause early morning insomnia • Can cause memory disturbances ("Traveler's amnesia" and anterograde amnesia) • Can cause daytime anxiety • Additive effects with alcohol and CNS depressants • Rare, unpredictable, idiosyncratic behavioral disturbances
• Free of residual side effects Suitable for initial insomnia • No accumulation • No withdrawal • Does not suppress REM sleep Minimal rebound insomnia • Delayed tolerance • Rapid onset	• Not available in Canada
Rapid onset Suitable for initial, middle, and late insomnia No accumulation • Delayed tolerance Minimal rebound insomnia Minimal interaction with alcohol and CNS depressants Minimal or no daytime anxiety No significant drug interactions Low side-effect profile Increased slow-wave sleep Does not suppress REM sleep	• Taste alteration • Not available in U.S.A.

has become a concern, especially with Triazolam.

The most commonly used benzodiazepines are listed on page 110. The main differences lie in the onset and duration of action. Understanding these mechanisms is important in the selection of the appropriate hypnotic drug for short and long term use.

Benzodiazepines are absorbed rapidly and almost completely from the intestinal tract. The onset of action usually begins within half an hour to five hours and the duration of action varies from a short two hours with Triazolam to 100 hours with Flurazepam.

Benzodiazepines are inactivated in the liver. Therefore, people with liver diseases, e.g., alcohol or viral hepatitis, will feel more side effects. Food and antacids slow the rate of absorption of benzodiazepines. With benzodiazepines, total sleep time is increased, sleep onset is quicker, and the number and duration of awakenings at night are significantly reduced.

In patients with insomnia, nonREM Stage I sleep is increased. With benzodiazepines, Stage I sleep is significantly decreased. Stage II sleep is increased, but Stages III and IV sleep (deep sleep) are generally decreased. REM sleep is usually suppressed.

The selection of benzodiazepines depends on the type of insomnia, e.g., inability to fall asleep or inability to maintain sleep, or both, and on the desired daytime effect.

The most common adverse effects of benzodiazepines are daytime sedation, rebound insomnia, and anterograte amnesia. Anxiety during the night is a major problem with very short acting drugs.

Daytime sedation is directly related to the dose, half- life of the drug, and development of tolerance to a drug.

Rebound insomnia depends on the half life of the drug. It is insomnia that occurs with abrupt withdrawal of the drug and is most common with the ultrashort acting drugs, e.g., Triazolam. Smaller doses with slow withdrawal may be the answer. The longer acting drugs, e.g., Flurazepam, generally produce mild rebound insomnia.

Non-Benzodiazepine Hypnotics: Zopiclone (Imovane) and Zolpidem (Stillnox, Ambien) are the two newest hypnotic medications. Although they bind to the benzodiazepine receptor, they bind to different portions or sub-units. The result is more specific sleep promoting properties, improved sleep quality, very little tolerance or dependence potential and fewer undesirable side effects. Zopiclone does not suppress REM sleep and may increase deep sleep. This latter effect may take three to four weeks (in some patients up to two months) to develop. For this reason a period of four to eight weeks on this medication is occasionally recommended to promote development of a good quality of sleep.

"Natural" Hypnotics

Tryptophan is an essential amino acid. It is weakly hypnotic and may accentuate the beneficial effect of antidepressants (chapter 4).

Melatonin is a naturally occurring hormone released during sleep. It has been shown to significantly improve sleep in some chronic insomniacs. It is thought to provide important information to the brain regarding time of day and of year.

Phenothiazine Antipsychotics

These drugs do not have primary effects on sleep, but they tend to decrease wakefulness and increase sleep time. They should not usually be used for insomnia, except in psychotic or mentally agitated people who need a sedative effect. The side effects of these drugs limit their usefullness as sleeping aids.

Sedative Tricyclic Antidepressants

These drugs including amitriptyline, doxepine, trimipramine, trazodone, clomipramine are used to treat depression not insomnia. They help reduce the depression and the insomnias in depressed people.

Most of these drugs reduce REM sleep and nightmares may be a problem on withdrawal. Clomipramine (Anafranil) is used to suppress nightmares.

Many different drugs can be used in treating insomnia. These are the general rules to follow.

• Use a drug made for this purpose.

• Usually take a drug for three to four weeks. Longer use could lead to an exacerbation of other causes of insomnia.

• A course of sleep medication is best, i.e., continuous use over a few weeks, rather than irregular dosing (an exception would be in treating jet lag, for example). If you know in advance that you are taking a course of treatment to improve sleep quality and quantity, it is usually easier to stop taking the drug at the end of a month. This helps with withdrawal and provides another chance to look at the cause of the insomnia if it persists beyond the month.

• Used well, sleeping medications are very helpful. Doctors who state that they never use sleeping pills are using neither the art nor the science of medicine.

• Drugs that are more specific and do not alter sleep architecture are preferable.

Following these general guidelines, you can use sleeping pills to complement the behavioral and other techniques previously discussed.

CHAPTER TWENTY-TWO

Another Sleep Diary

I n preceding chapters we have presented a wide array of possible interventions that may help you improve your sleep. We emphasized at the beginning of this section that you should not attempt too many changes at once. We hope that you have tried over several weeks to introduce three or four of the most crucial changes that might have addressed your sleep disruption. If perhaps you were too wound up before getting into bed, or, when you were in bed, worried about the various activities of the day, you have, by now, adopted a pattern of regular relaxation, and perhaps effected a "thought stopping" technique. This combination of activities is like trying to make a left hand turn while driving a car fast. What one needs to do first is to slow down the car and then make the turn. The relaxation technique has been the application of the brakes. Once that has been done, it is possible to change the pattern of thoughts going through the mind.

If your problem relates to long-term use of sleeping pills or unnecessary consumption of alcohol leading to disrupted sleep, you will have hopefully changed in your behavior. You may have also gone to your family physician or another professional for help.

In acquiring any behavioral skill (and in large measure, sleep is a learned behavior in which practice improves performance) one has to go through the process of making changes and checking their effectiveness. A tennis player learning new strokes or techniques practices them specifically and then puts them into the context of his or her game.

Perhaps the severity of your insomnia has led you to your doctor who has prescribed a course of hypnotics. Often insomniacs are better able to make necessary behavioral changes while taking sleeping tablets. When the period on medication ends, the behavioral improvements allow for continued good sleep.

We suggest that while continuing to use the techniques you have chosen you again make a one-week evaluation of your sleep routine, behavioral activities, and subjective feelings using the *new diary* on pages 116 and 117. This is a rerun of your earlier assessment. The most important part of this exercise is that you stick to it and that you report the information accurately.

Now you can compare the *new* ratings with the *old*. There should be a substantive difference. For most patients going through this exercise when directed by a physician, there will be dramatic change. If there is, you should persist with the techniques you have developed and the changes in lifestyle you have instituted to improve your sleep quality. If there is no clear change, it may be that you have misidentified some of the key issues, or that we have been unable to guide you to the specific cause of your sleep disruption. It may be that something fairly obvious has, in fact, been recorded, but because it is so inherent in your lifestyle it is difficult for you to see it as a problem.

We have often used some of these techniques with groups of patients with insomnia. Occasionally, individuals will fill out their own sleep diary and will not be able to see any fault in their behavior patterns. We ask a pair of patients to swap diaries and each is quite able to see the faults in the behaviors of the other but not in his own. It may be helpful to take along this manual when consulting your physician or a sleep specialist so they may review the information you have so carefully collected about yourself. They may identify problems that you have not been able to recognize.

Insomnia can recur. A patient on long-term benzodiazepine medication who withdrew by using the drug Zopiclone and then instituted behavioral techniques, remained off medication for ten months, only to develop severe insomnia and require medication again when a close friend was diagnosed with breast cancer and faced death. Re-initiation of the behavioral techniques that had been helpful before, together with brief use of medication, allowed for a quick improvement of sleep.

It is important to remember that these techniques are perfected with practice. To think that if you suddenly have one bad night you will be able to simply switch on a relaxation skill is not realistic. However, if you have acquired a tape cassette or previously practiced behavioral skills, or have found previous pharmacological treatments helpful on a short-term basis, then you will find similar help easier to obtain. The result will be a good sleep and a feeling of being well-rested which will allow you to tackle the day with vigor.

"Come, Sleep! O Sleep, the certain knot of peace,
The baiting-place of wit, the balm of woe,
The poor man's wealth, the prisoner's release,
Th' indifferent judge between the high and low."

(*Sir Philip Sidney, 1554-1586,* Astrophel and Stella)

SLEEP AND ACTIVITIES RECORD

Instructions: It is important that you fill out this chart each evening
Mark your diary in the following way

ACTIVITIES
A - each alcoholic drink
C - each caffeinated drink: includes coffee, tea, chocolate, cola
I   - interaction of calmness. This may be an exciting movie on TV, sexual
    intercourse before sleeping, a noise during sleep, or anxious thoughts
P - every time you take a sleeping pill or tranquilizer
P2 - every time you take any other pill
M - meals
S - snacks
X - exercise
T - use of toilet during sleep time

SLEEP TIME (including naps)
D - lights out/dark
I   - lights on/illumination
B - alarm clock wakening

Note each entry to bed with ↓
Note each exit from bed with ↑
Note time asleep with ⊢——⊣

NOON	2	4	6	8	10	MIDNIGHT	2	4	6	8	10	NOON

n the assessment of performance we would like you to use the scale from 0 to 0. For example, you might record a 1 or 2 if you are very sleepy, but if very efreshed, you would record an 8 or 9. This page is divided into two parts, hose features that should be recorded 15 to 20 minutes after "arising" (A, B, :, D, E) and those items to be recorded before bedtime (1, 2, 3).

WAKE - ZZZ CHART

emember to complete A-E approximately 15 -20 minutes after awakening.
omplete 1-3 prior to switching off your light at night.

				Very Sleepy 0 1 2 3 4 5 6 7 8 9 10 Fully refreshed			
	Morning				**Evening**		
Fill in date under day	A	B	C	D	E	1	2	3
	Hours of sleep last night	I awoke very sleepy = 0; very refresh-ed = 10	I feel fuzzy headed = 0; alert = 10	My sleep was restless = 0; tranquil = 10	My sleep was better than usual = 0; as usual = 5; very dis-rupted = 10	I feel very tired = 0; wide awake = 10	I feel phys-ically worn out = 0; re-laxed = 10	I feel tense = 0; calm = 10
Monday								
Tuesday								
Wednesday								
Thursday								
Friday								
Saturday								
Sunday								

APPENDIX

The following addresses may be helpful in obtaining informatio about various aspects of sleep.

World Federation of Sleep Societies
Dr. Michael Chase, President, c/o Brain Information Service, UCL School of Medicine, Los Angeles, California, USA 90024-174(Telephone (310) 825-3417, Telefax (310) 206-3499

The World Federation of Sleep Research Societies (WFSRS) an international association of sleep research societies aimed i promoting sleep studies worldwide and at strengthening inte national relations among sleep researchers and clinicians. There a a number of member societies, for example, the Canadian Slee Society and the European Sleep Research Society. If you wa information about a local sleep society as a contact point to obtai details about local research or the names of clinicians who treat slee disorders, the WFSRS may be able to help.

National Sleep Foundation
Mrs. Carol Westbrook, Executive Director, 122 South Robertsc Blvd., Third Floor, Los Angeles, California, USA 90048. Telephon (310) 288-0466, Telefax (310) 288-0570

The National Sleep Foundation is a non-profit charitable o ganization established to help improve the quality of life t promoting knowledge about sleep, its disorders, and its relation t health. The Foundation serves as a national referral service an coordinating center for public information.

Sleep/Wake Disorders Canada
Mrs. Bev Devins, 3089 Bathurst St., Suite 304, Toronto, Ontari(Canada M6A 2A4. Telephone (416) 787-5374, Toll-Free 1-800-387-925. Telefax (416) 787-4431

Sleep/Wake Disorders Canada is a non-profit volunteer cha itable association which encourages and supports anyone with ar type of sleep disorder. Non-professional members facilitate self-hel groups and provide support. Its members work to improve th quality of life, alertness, and productivity of persons with sleep/wak disorders.

Sleep Devices Inc.
Mr. Kevin O'Donnell, P.O. Box 23510, Dexter P.O., 5899 Leslie St Willowdale, Ontario, Canada, M2H 3R9. Telephone (416) 889-646(Telefax (416) 889-3649

This is a mail order business dedicated to providing a range (sleep-related appliances including anti-snoring devices, anti-alle genic bedding, video material, relaxation tapes, and light therar equipment.

GLOSSARY

anorexia nervosa - an eating disorder in which people avoid eating and lose weight, but may continue to perceive themselves as being fat even if they are thin.

anterograde amnesia - a loss of short term memory for events immediately preceding a trauma.

apnea - a cessation of breathing.

biological clock - an internal body clock which controls the rhythms of sleep and wakefulness, hormones, and temperature.

bright-light phototherapy - a treatment, employing special lights, used for people with winter depression which may be helpful in certain types of insomnia as well.

calorimetry - measurement of the body's energy expenditure (metabolism).

carpal tunnel syndrome - pain and weakness of the palm of the hand caused by entrapment of the median nerve at the wrist.

cholecystokinin - an enzyme released by the pancreas which causes contraction of the gall bladder to release stored bile.

chronic fatigue syndrome - a syndrome characterized by at least six months of exceptional fatigue, with greater than 50 percent reduction in activity level.

circadian rhythm - internal changes (e.g., in temperature) which follow a cycle of approximately 24 hours and are synchronized, to some extent, by external factors such as light and dark.

diurnal - daily

enuresis - inability to keep bladder control.

extrinsic (sleep disorders) - external factors such as light or temperature which affect sleep.

fibromyalgia - chronic diffuse musculoskeletal soreness, aching, and tenderness, usually accompanied by tiredness, sleep disruption, and non-restorative sleep. There must also be pain in 11 of 18 tender points on digital palpitation.

fibrositis - a common form of rheumatism characterized by generalized muscle aches and tender points in soft tissue.

glaucoma (acute angle closure) - a condition of the eye

characterized by extreme pain, redness, blurred vision, and a dilated non-reactive pupil. Treatment must be sought within 12 - 48 hours or blindness may occur.

hyperventilation - excessive breathing.

hypoglycemic coma - coma due to very low blood sugar levels.

intrinsic (sleep disorders) - internal events such as hormone levels which affect sleep.

MSLT - Multiple Sleep Latency Test

MWT - Maintenance of Wakefulness Test

myocardial infarction - destruction of the heart muscle by inadequate blood supply.

narcolepsy - a disorder characterized by frequent and irresistible daytime sleepiness, hallucinations, and full or partial paralysis.

nocturnal - pertaining to the night; active at night.

nocturnal myoclonus - muscle cramps, especially of calf muscles occurring at night.

phase delay - disruption to the circadian rhythm which results in biological events, such as sleep onset, occurring later than normal.

PMR - Progressive Muscle Relaxation

restless legs syndrome - disagreeable leg sensations leading to an irresistible urge to move the legs which brings relief from the sensations.

SAD - seasonal affective disorder

sleep state misperception - a belief that one has had little or no sleep when the facts are otherwise.

stress - stress exists when the adaptive capacity of the person is overwhelmed by events.

SCN (Suprachiasmatic nucleus) - a part of the brain that controls biological rhythms.

Yerkes-Dodson Curve - a curve that shows the relation of stress to performance (Figure 9-1).